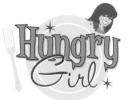

FAST
& easy

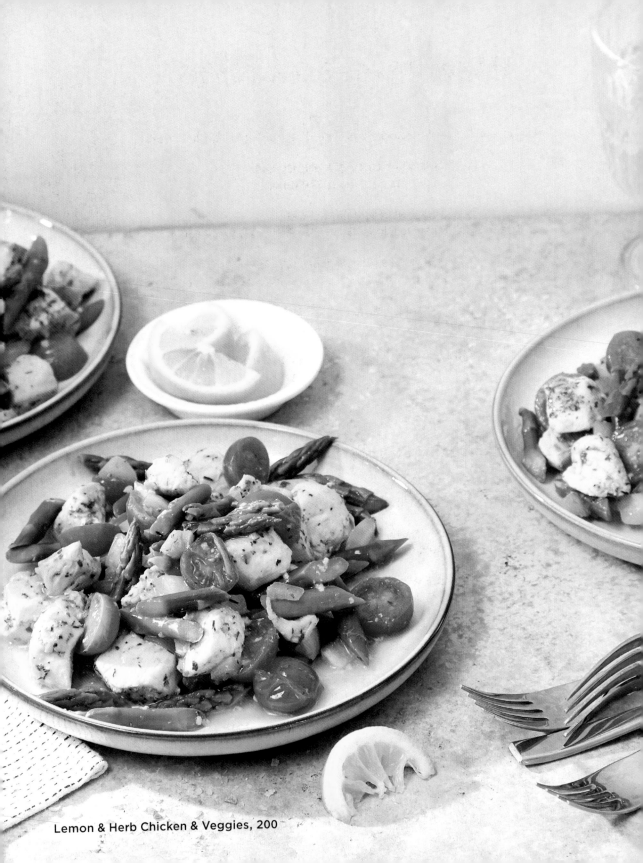

Lemon & Herb Chicken & Veggies, 200

Also by Lisa Lillien

HUNGRY GIRL:
Recipes and Survival Strategies for Guilt-Free Eating in the Real World

HUNGRY GIRL 200 UNDER 200:
200 Recipes Under 200 Calories

HUNGRY GIRL 1-2-3:
The Easiest, Most Delicious, Guilt-Free Recipes on the Planet

HUNGRY GIRL HAPPY HOUR:
75 Recipes for Amazingly Fantastic Guilt-Free Cocktails & Party Foods

HUNGRY GIRL 300 UNDER 300:
300 Breakfast, Lunch & Dinner Dishes Under 300 Calories

HUNGRY GIRL SUPERMARKET SURVIVAL:
Aisle by Aisle, HG-Style!

HUNGRY GIRL TO THE MAX!
The Ultimate Guilt-Free Cookbook

HUNGRY GIRL 200 UNDER 200 JUST DESSERTS:
200 Recipes Under 200 Calories

THE HUNGRY GIRL DIET

THE HUNGRY GIRL DIET COOKBOOK:
Healthy Recipes for Mix-n-Match Meals & Snacks

HUNGRY GIRL CLEAN & HUNGRY:
Easy All-Natural Recipes for Healthy Eating in the Real World

HUNGRY GIRL CLEAN & HUNGRY OBSESSED!
All-Natural Recipes for the Foods You Can't Live Without

HUNGRY GIRL SIMPLY 6:
All-Natural Recipes with 6 Ingredients or Less

HUNGRY GIRL: THE OFFICIAL SURVIVAL GUIDES:
Tips & Tricks for Guilt-Free Eating
(audio book)

HUNGRY GIRL CHEW THE RIGHT THING:
Supreme Makeovers for 50 Foods You Crave
(recipe cards)

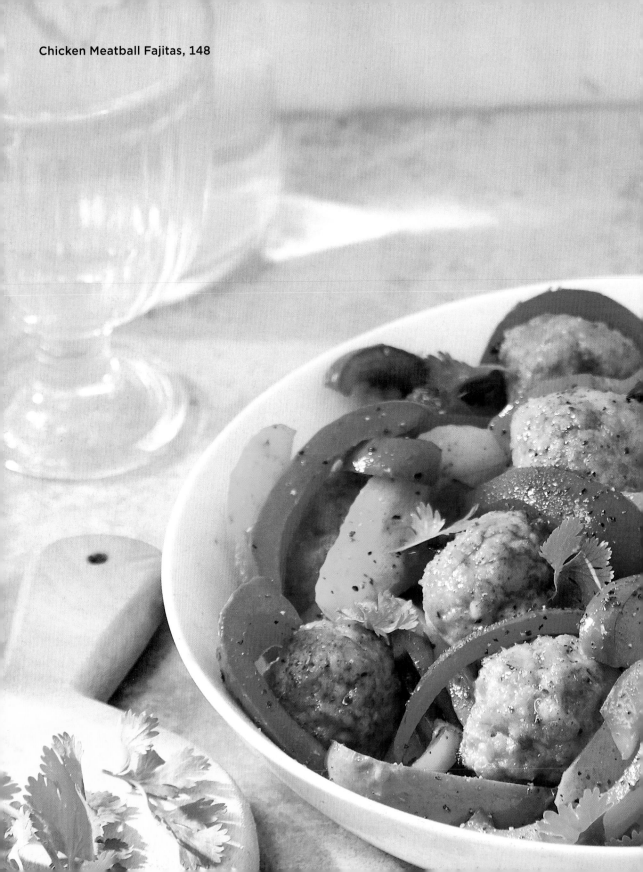

Chicken Meatball Fajitas, 148

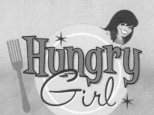

FAST & easy

All-Natural Recipes in 30 Minutes or Less

LISA LILLIEN

St. Martin's Griffin
New York

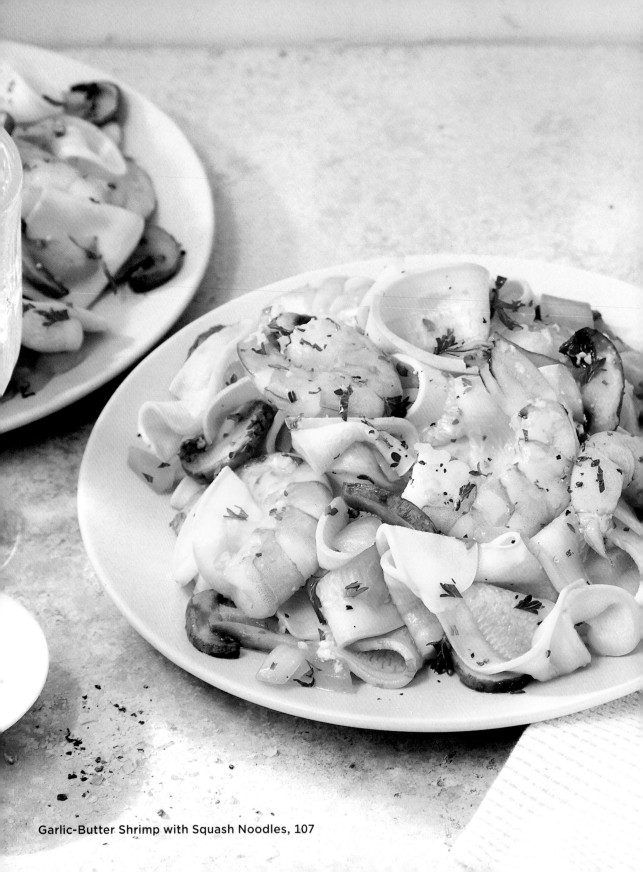

Garlic-Butter Shrimp with Squash Noodles, 107

Get More
Hungry Girl

For the latest better-for-you recipes, food finds, healthy-eating tips & tricks, and MORE . . .

✉ **Sign up for FREE daily emails** at hungry-girl.com

Follow Lisa on Facebook at facebook.com/hungrygirl

Join the Hungry Girl Community: What's Chewin'? group on Facebook

Follow Lisa on Instagram . . . She's @hungrygirl

Listen to the *Hungry Girl: Chew the Right Thing!* podcast at hungry-girl.com/podcast

Check out Hungry Girl on Pinterest at pinterest.com/hungrygirl

First published in the United States by St. Martin's Griffin, an imprint of St. Martin's Publishing Group

www.stmartins.com

Cover design by Lisa Yager and Ralph Fowler
Book design by Ralph Fowler
Illustrations by Jack Pullan
Food styling by Marian Cooper Cairns
Food photography by Jennifer Davick

The Library of Congress Cataloging-in-Publication Data is available upon request.

ISBN 9781250154545 (trade paperback)
ISBN 9781250154552 (ebook)

Our books may be purchased in bulk for promotional, educational, or business use. Please contact your local bookseller or the Macmillan Corporate and Premium Sales Department at 1-800-221-7945, extension 5442, or by email at MacmillanSpecialMarkets@macmillan.com.

First Edition: 2021

10 9 8 7 6 5 4 3 2 1

This book is dedicated to the memory of my sweet & lovable pepperoni-pizza-loving pal Leah Bernstein, and all my other friends from MPTF's Mary Pickford House who lost their battles with COVID-19 last Spring. You are missed.

Contents

1

Salads & Slaws

Poultry

Beef & Pork

Seafood

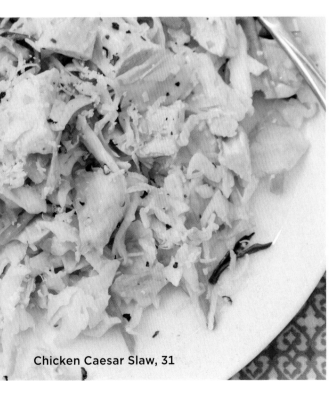

Chicken Caesar Slaw, 31

2

Stir-Frys & Skillet Meals

Poultry

Beef & Pork

Seafood

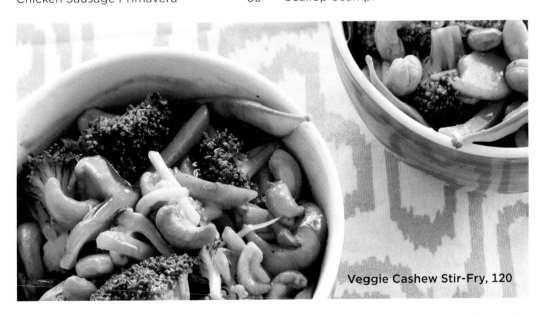

Veggie Cashew Stir-Fry, 120

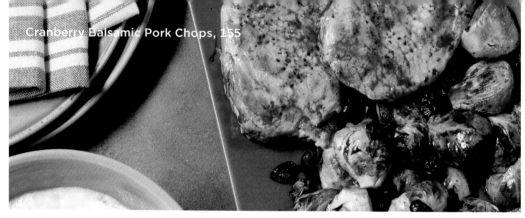

Cranberry Balsamic Pork Chops, 155

Sheet-Pan Meals

Poultry

Beef & Pork

Seafood

Meatless

4

One-Pot Recipes

Poultry

Beef & Pork

Seafood

Meatless

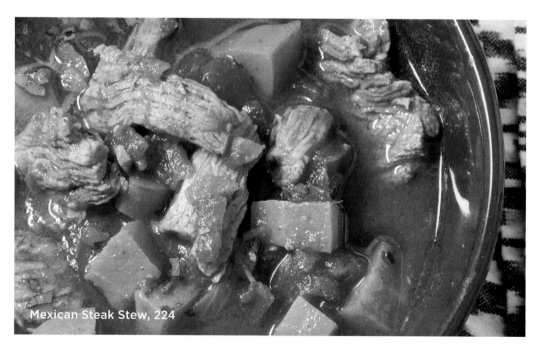

Mexican Steak Stew, 224

10-Minute Power Bowls

5-Minute Salad Dressings

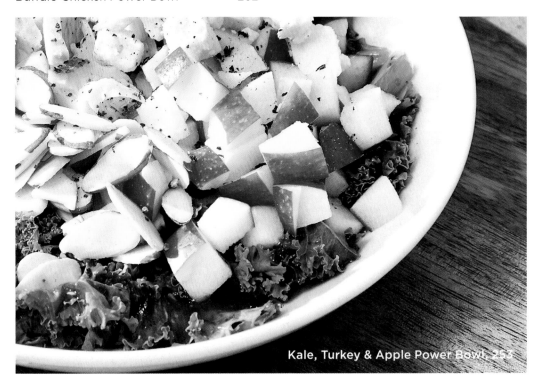

Kale, Turkey & Apple Power Bowl, 253

3-Ingredient Protein Rollups

Speedy Cucumber Subs

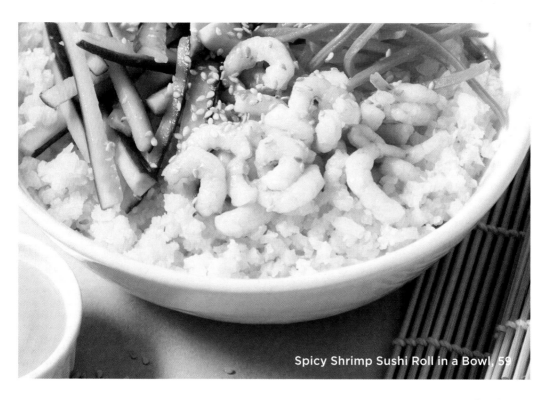

Spicy Shrimp Sushi Roll in a Bowl, 59

9

5-Minute Smoothies

10

Quickie Crepes

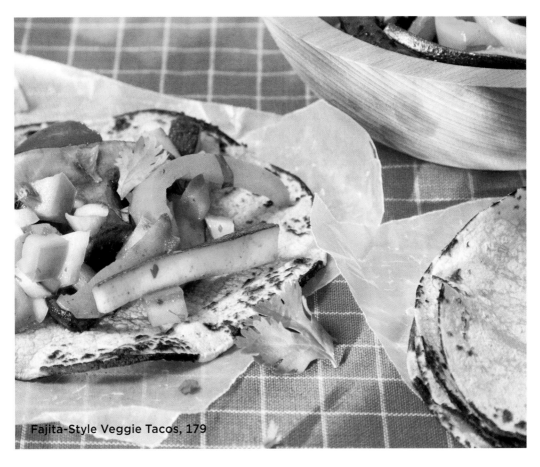

Fajita-Style Veggie Tacos, 179

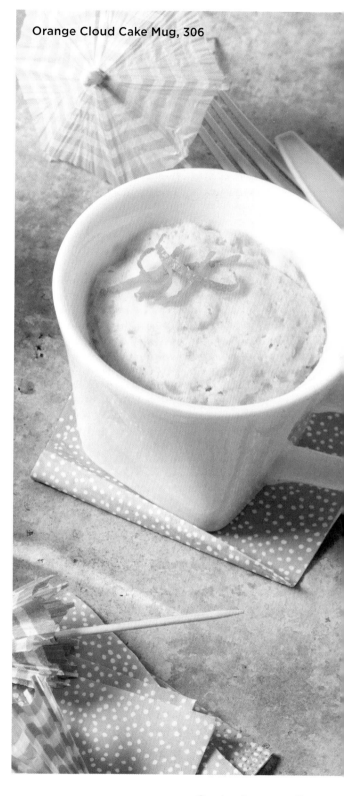
Orange Cloud Cake Mug, 306

2-Ingredient Cake Mugs

Fast & Easy Kitchen Guides

Acknowledgments

Recipe books don't just appear out of nowhere. Not even ones that are this *fast & easy*. The following folks deserve huge kudos and tremendous thank-yous . . .

Jamie Goldberg—Thanks once again for being a dream to work with, a creative dynamo, and the master of keeping everyone and everything (including me!) in line. You are truly the strong nuclear force that holds all the subatomic particles of our team together.

The better-than-ever Hungry Girl book team—you are all INCREDIBLE!
Lynn Bettencourt
Dana DeRuyck
Erin Norcross
Katie Killeavy
Lydia Oxenham

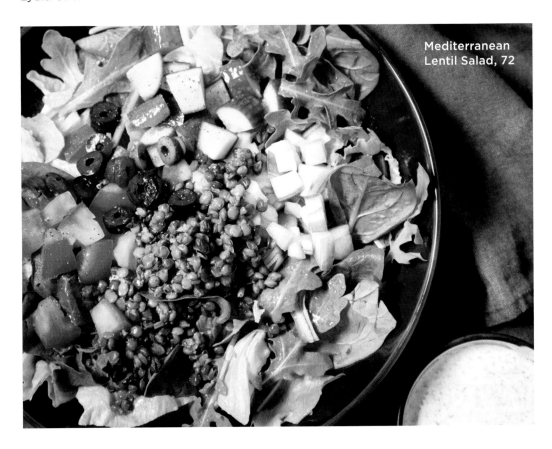

Mediterranean
Lentil Salad, 72

Special thanks to these wonderful Hungry Girl team members for all they do . . .
Peggy Mansfield
Gina Muscato
Mike Sherry
Olga Gatica

And to my extended HG family . . .
John Vaccaro
Neeti Madan
Jennifer Enderlin
John Karle
Anne Marie Tallberg
Brant Janeway
Erica Martirano
Elizabeth Catalano
Sallie Lotz
James Sinclair
Lena Shekhter
Tracey Guest
Bill Stankey
Tom Fineman
Steve Younger
Jeff Becker
Susan Garcia
Ruby Magsambol
Lauren Lillien
Amanda Maisonet

These creative humans deserve thanks for making the book so beautiful . . .
Ralph Fowler
Jennifer Davick
Marian Cooper Cairns
Jack Pullan

And, as always, endless gratitude and love to my family . . .
Daniel Schneider
Florence and Maurice Lillien
Meri Lillien
Jay Lillien
Lolly, Bam Bam and Jordan

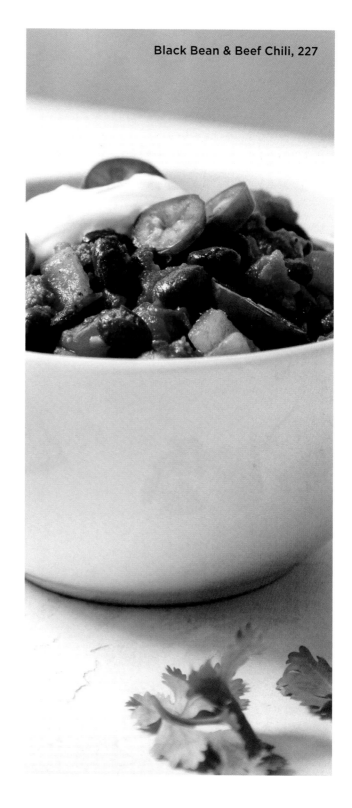

Black Bean & Beef Chili, 227

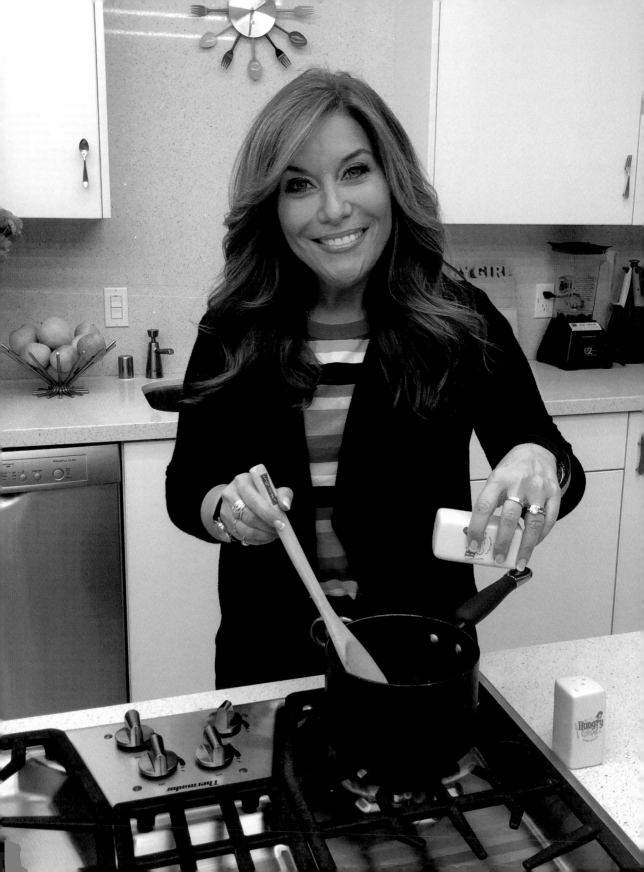

Hi!

Lisa here, and I can't believe I am writing an introduction for my FOURTEENTH book. It's crazy to think that I started Hungry Girl almost seventeen years ago and have been cranking out fun, delicious, and simple recipes ever since. My goal has always been to keep things easy, while serving up big portions of better-for-you food that tastes great! I love what I do so much—and I continue to feel inspired and excited to learn, grow, and share more creations with the world!

When it comes to cookbooks, I've pretty much done it all . . . recipes under 200 calories, ones under 300 calories, cocktail and party recipes, clean recipes, meals with six (or fewer!) main ingredients, and so much more. And with each book, I truly feel that the recipes get better and better. But if there's one thing I've learned over the last few years it's that people are cooking more at home—but they really want to spend less time doing it. So I decided to take things one step further on the simplicity scale and bring you a collection of super speedy and delicious meals that take 30 minutes or less to make—salads, slaws, skillet meals, sheet-pan meals, one-pot meals, and more! As an added bonus, I've included dozens of recipes for sweet treats, salad dressings, smoothies, and snacks!

I'm actually surprised it's taken me this long to bring you a book of 30-minute meals because I am one of the most impatient people ever. I don't like waiting for things—especially food. When I was a little kid, I would often be seen sneaking food out of pots and pans during the final cooking stages of dinner. (Sorry, Mom!) And this is not something I'm proud of, but I would occasionally snack on my favorite freezer-aisle chicken drummies with icy centers because 45 minutes was simply too long to wait for 'em! (Not my most impressive moment.) Eventually, I grew up enough to learn that good food often takes time—but luckily (and as evidenced by this fine publication) it doesn't have to take a lot of it.

Now I know if you're holding this book in your hands, you're probably more interested in diving in and whipping up something delicious than reading more words from me (no matter how entertaining I attempt to make them)! So without further delay . . . I present to you . . . *HUNGRY GIRL FAST & EASY!*

Happy chewing!!!
Lisa :)

FAQs

Who & what is Hungry Girl?

It's me, Lisa Lillien (a.k.a. Hungry Girl)! I'm not a nutritionist. I'm just hungry. I don't have any fancy medical degrees, but I do consider myself a "foodologist," because I love finding easy and healthy ways to eat delicious food . . . and a LOT of it!

Hungry Girl began in 2004 as a daily email that I sent to my friends and family. Today, millions of fans access Hungry Girl content via the free daily emails (sign up at hungry-girl.com), my social media pages, *Hungry Girl* magazine, the HG podcast, and more. My goal has always been to help people eat better and achieve their weight-management goals in a fun, real-world way. And *Fast & Easy* does exactly that!

What makes these recipes fast & easy?

Each and every one of these recipes takes 30 minutes or LESS from start to finish. That means in the time it takes to watch a sitcom, you can whip up a healthy & delicious meal. In fact, many of these recipes only take 10 minutes!

That's the fast part. Here's the easy part: Each recipe calls for just a few simple, everyday ingredients. No mile-long ingredient lists. No organic lavender petals. (That's a thing, right?) Just healthy grocery staples and easy-to-follow directions!

What makes them all natural?

These recipes mostly call for "whole" natural ingredients: think lean protein, fruit, veggies, eggs, and more. Any other ingredients—like cheese, condiments, or canned goods—are readily available in stores without anything artificial added. When in doubt, look for trusted natural brands or shop at a natural foods store.

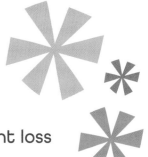

Are these recipes good for weight loss or meant for a specific diet?

When it comes to Hungry Girl recipes, the goal is always to have something completely satisfying with impressive nutritional stats. Most of these recipes are high in protein & fiber, and low in starchy carbs, added sugars, and calories. They won't magically make you lose weight, but they'll fill you up without weighing you down, and they fit perfectly into many weight-loss plans.

Now, as a "foodologist" (remember, I'm not a nutrition professional), I don't offer medical advice related to dietary conditions. But what I do provide is full nutritional information carefully calculated for each and every recipe. I'm giving you the tools to work these low-calorie recipes into your personal lifestyle or diet plan. Feel free to modify them and make them work for you!

Where can I find the WW points values?

There are lots of WW fans in the Hungry Girl universe! To support anyone on a WW journey, we calculate the points values for all Hungry Girl recipes. At WW's request, and because the points system changes from time to time, we don't include these values in Hungry Girl cookbooks. But we DO provide the recipe values online. Visit hungry-girl.com/fast&easy for the WW points values* of the recipes in this book.

*SmartPoints® values for these recipes were calculated by Hungry Girl and are not an endorsement or approval of the recipe or its developer by WW International, Inc., the owner of the SmartPoints® trademark.

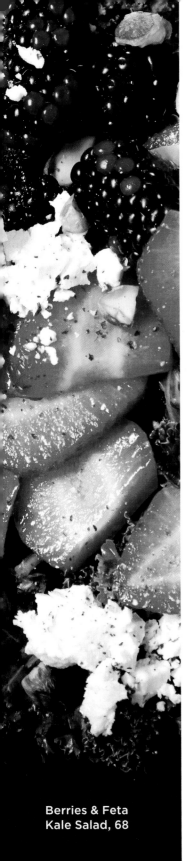

Berries & Feta
Kale Salad, 68

Fast & Easy Recipe Guide

Gluten-free, vegetarian, no-cook . . . *Fast & Easy* has it all! Look for the following symbols on each recipe, or check out the guides on the following pages.

NC   No-Cook Recipes

5i   Recipes with 5 Ingredients or Less

15m   Recipes in 15 Minutes or Less

30m   Recipes in 30 Minutes or Less

V   Vegetarian Recipes

GF   Gluten-Free Recipes

Pssst . . . Don't miss the BONUS lists for single-serving and family-size recipes!

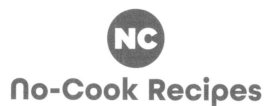

No-Cook Recipes

Keep your cool . . . You don't need your oven, stove, or microwave for these recipes.

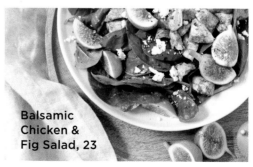

Balsamic Chicken & Fig Salad, 23

Recipes with 5 Ingredients or Less

It's true . . . Each of these recipes has no more than five main ingredients! (Basic seasonings, ice, and water don't count.)

Recipes in 15 Minutes or Less

Speedy salads, 10-minute power bowls, 5-minute smoothies . . .
Over 75 recipes in just 15 minutes or less!

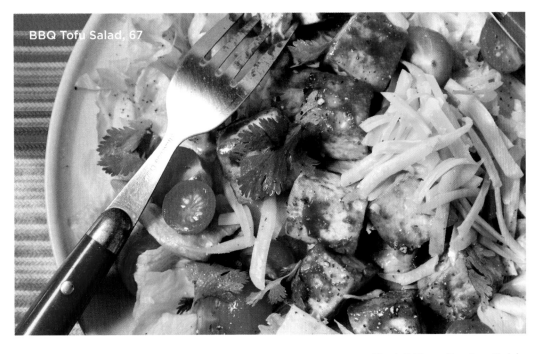

BBQ Tofu Salad, 67

Recipes in 30 Minutes or Less

EVERY recipe in this cookbook takes half an hour max to make. These recipes are ready in 20 to 30 minutes . . .

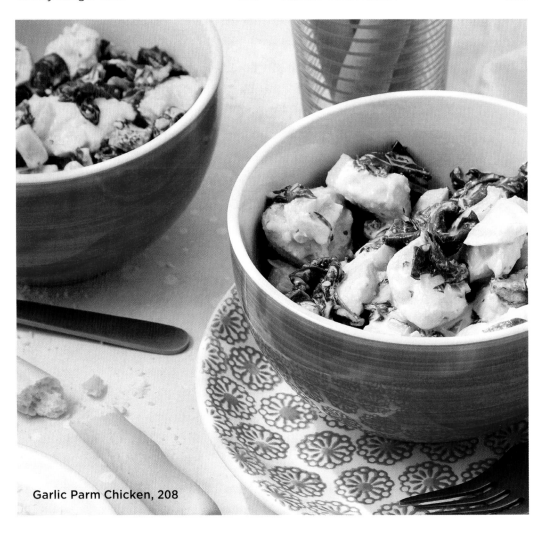

Garlic Parm Chicken, 208

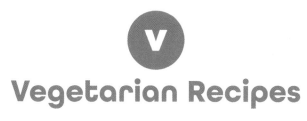

Vegetarian Recipes

No red meat, poultry, seafood, or animal by-products are found in these recipes. They aren't all vegan (they may include dairy or eggs), but I'm offering up plant-based ingredient swaps on page 320!

Gluten-Free Recipes

Wowowowow . . . 100+ recipes with no gluten in sight!

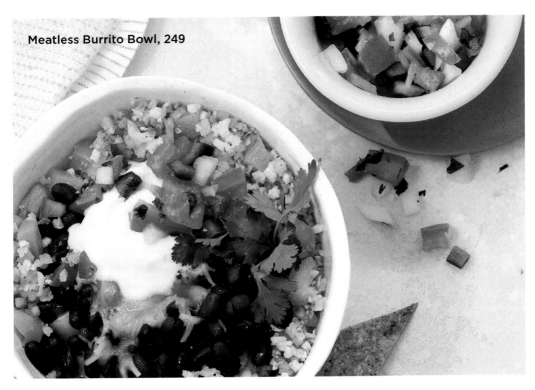

Meatless Burrito Bowl, 249

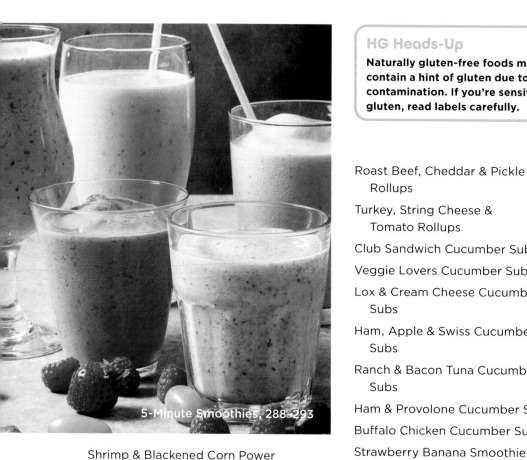

5-Minute Smoothies, 288–293

Single-Serve Recipes

Delicious meals for one . . . Coming right up!

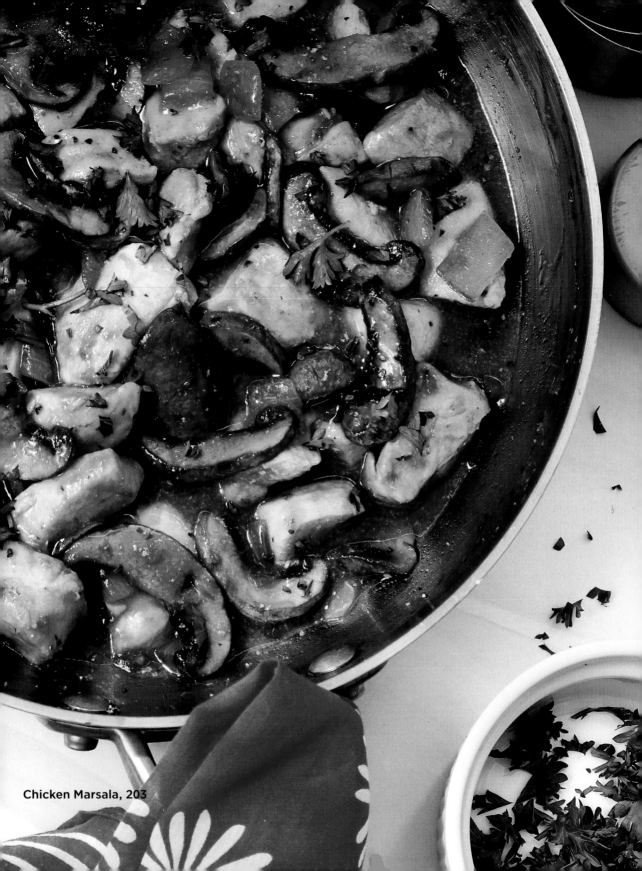

Chicken Marsala, 203

Family-Size Recipes

Feeding a crowd (or just enjoy having leftovers for days)?
Each of these recipes has four or more servings.

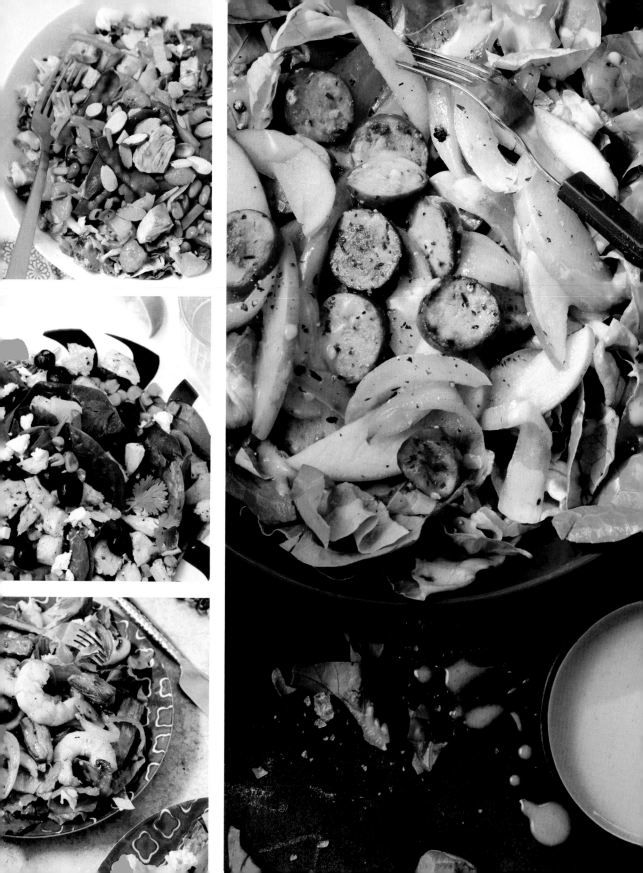

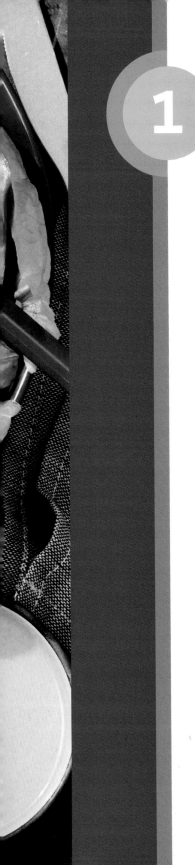

1

Salads & Slaws

Lettuce never looked so good. I've got cold salads, warm salads, and flavorful slaws . . . most of 'em ready in 15 minutes or less! Bonus: Flip to page 263 for 11 DIY salad dressings that are fast and flavor packed!

Chicken Souvlaki Salad

286 calories

Such a flavorful upgrade from regular grilled chicken salad! My dressing of choice: the Cucumber Feta Dressing on page 271.

Prep: 5 minutes

Cook: 10 minutes

You'll need:
large bowl, small bowl, skillet, nonstick spray

Entire recipe:
286 calories
10.5g total fat
(1.5g sat fat)
363mg sodium
21g carbs
5.5g fiber
13g sugars
28.5g protein

3 cups chopped lettuce
½ cup chopped cucumber
½ cup chopped tomato
1 tablespoon lemon juice
1½ teaspoons olive oil
1 teaspoon honey
⅛ teaspoon garlic powder
⅛ teaspoon dried oregano
4 ounces raw boneless skinless chicken breast, cut into bite-size pieces
¼ cup chopped red onion
⅛ teaspoon each salt and black pepper

1. Place lettuce in a large bowl. Top with cucumber and tomato.

2. To make the sauce, in a small bowl, combine lemon juice, oil, honey, garlic powder, and oregano. Add 1½ teaspoons water, and whisk with a fork until uniform.

3. Bring a skillet sprayed with nonstick spray to medium-high heat. Add chicken, onion, salt, pepper, and sauce. Cook and stir until chicken is fully cooked and onion has softened, about 5 minutes.

4. Spoon chicken mixture over the salad.

MAKES 1 SERVING

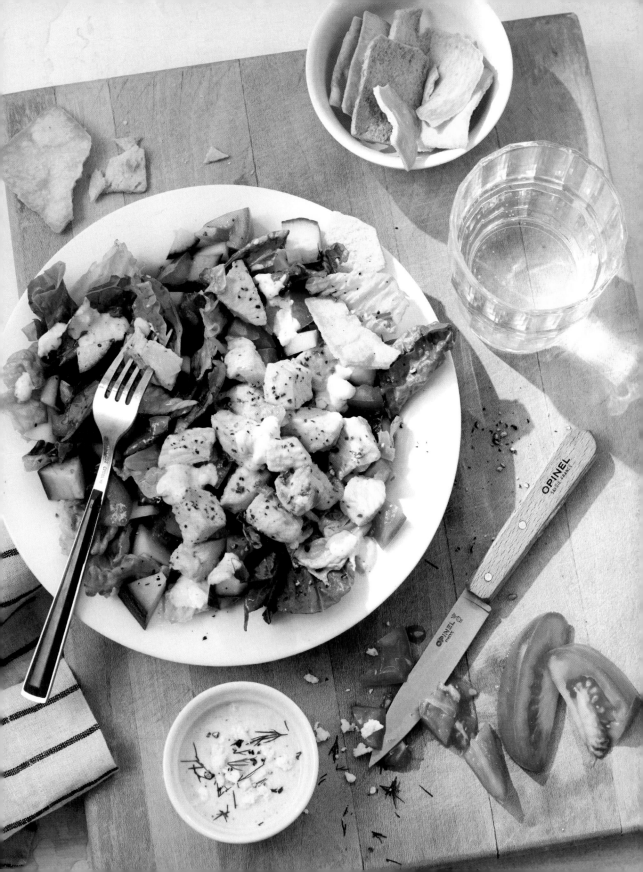

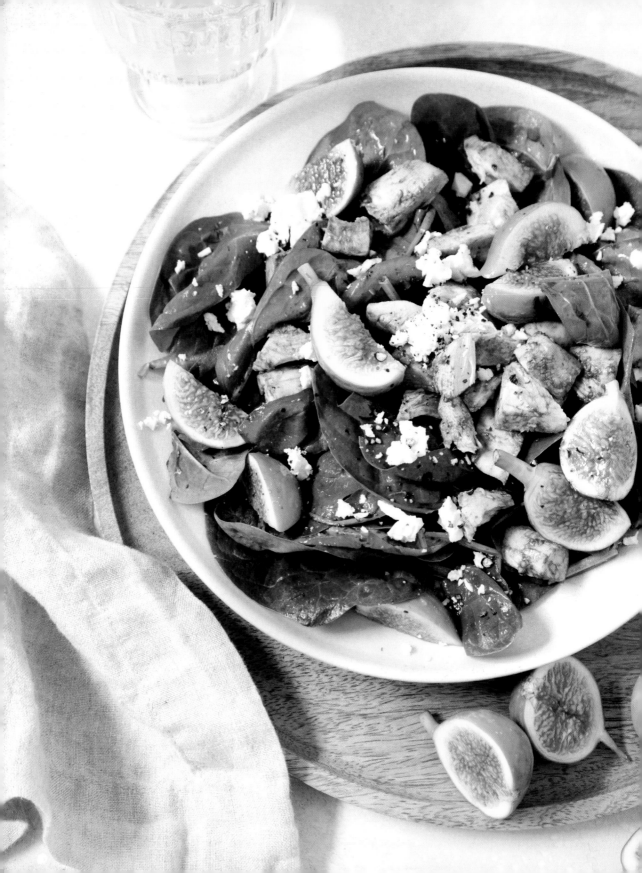

Balsamic Chicken & Fig Salad

3 cups spinach leaves

3 ounces cooked skinless chicken breast, cut into bite-size pieces

1 tablespoon balsamic vinegar

2 medium figs, sliced, or ¼ cup chopped dried figs

2 tablespoons crumbled feta cheese

1. Place spinach in a large bowl.

2. In a medium bowl, toss chicken with vinegar.

3. Spoon balsamic chicken over the spinach, and top with figs and feta.

MAKES 1 SERVING

280 calories

Prep: 5 minutes

You'll need:
large bowl,
medium bowl

Entire recipe:
280 calories
6.5g total fat
(3g sat fat)
295mg sodium
25g carbs
5g fiber
19g sugars
31g protein

HG FYI

Fresh figs are in season from late summer through early fall, but you can find dried figs year round at the supermarket where the raisins are stocked.

Salads & Slaws: Poultry

Warm Chinese Chicken Salad

341 calories

3 cups chopped lettuce

2 cups frozen stir-fry vegetables

3 ounces cooked skinless chicken breast, cut into bite-size pieces

2 tablespoons canned sliced water chestnuts, drained

1½ tablespoons thick teriyaki sauce or marinade

1 teaspoon chopped garlic

¼ teaspoon ground ginger

2 tablespoons mandarin orange segments packed in juice, drained and chopped

2 tablespoons chopped scallions

¼ ounce (about 1 tablespoon) sliced almonds

1. Place lettuce in a large bowl.

2. Bring a skillet sprayed with nonstick spray to medium-high heat. Add frozen veggies, cover, and cook for 3 minutes, or until thawed.

3. Add chicken, water chestnuts, teriyaki, garlic, and ginger to the skillet. Cook and stir until hot and well mixed, about 2 minutes.

4. Spoon chicken mixture over the lettuce, and top with orange segments, scallions, and almonds.

MAKES 1 SERVING

15m

Prep: 5 minutes

Cook: 10 minutes

You'll need:
large bowl, skillet with lid, nonstick spray

Entire recipe:
341 calories
7g total fat
(1g sat fat)
722mg sodium
34g carbs
8.5g fiber
16.5g sugars
32.5g protein

HG Tip
Grab some precooked chicken from the supermarket, or cook up a batch on the weekend to use all week.

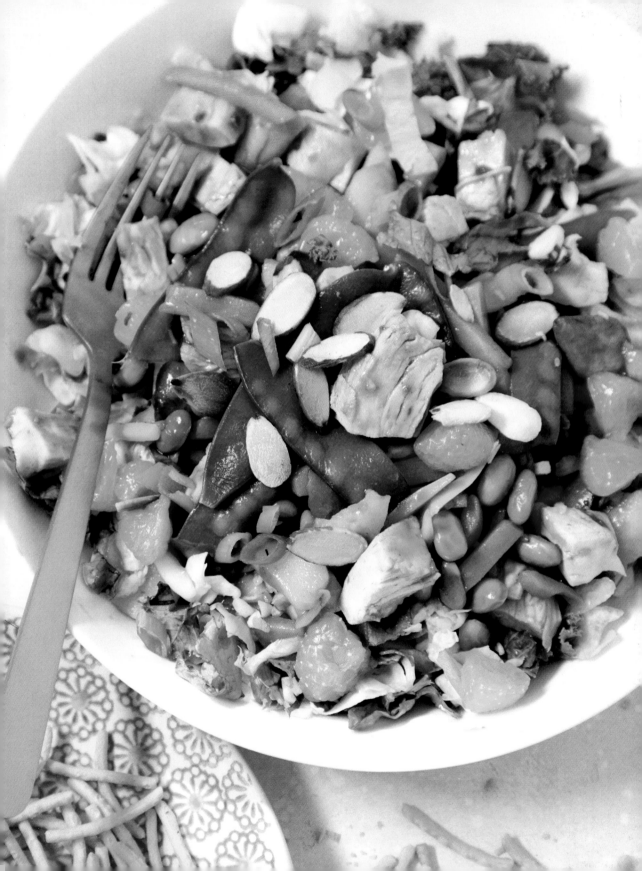

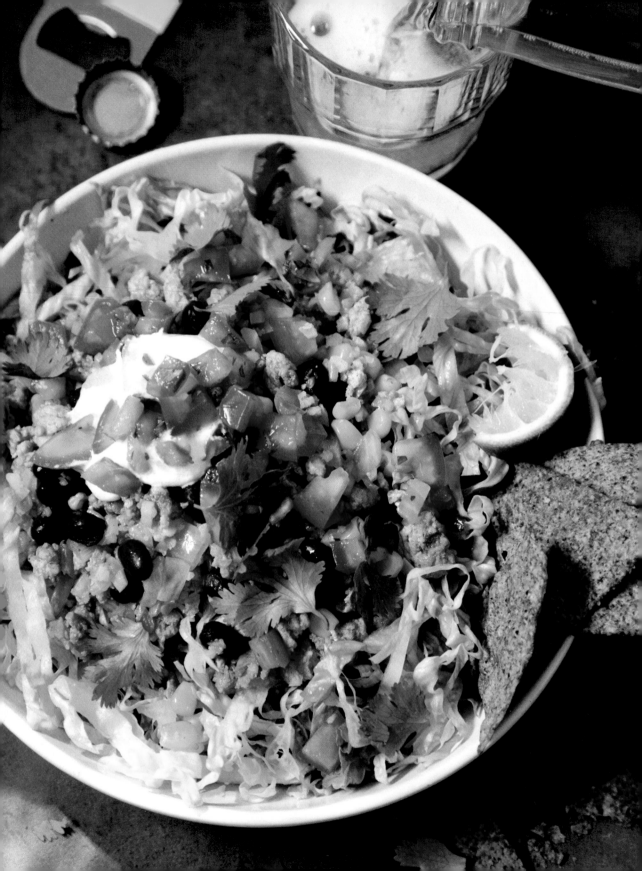

The cilantro is optional, but I highly recommend it.

3 cups shredded lettuce

4 ounces raw extra-lean ground chicken (at least 98% lean)

⅓ cup chopped onion

2 teaspoons taco seasoning

½ cup frozen riced cauliflower

¼ cup frozen sweet corn kernels

2 tablespoons canned black beans, drained and rinsed

2 tablespoons salsa

2 tablespoons light sour cream

Optional topping: chopped fresh cilantro

1. Place lettuce in a large bowl.

2. Bring a skillet sprayed with nonstick spray to medium-high heat. Add chicken, onion, and taco seasoning. Cook and crumble until chicken is fully cooked and onion has softened, about 5 minutes.

3. Add cauliflower and corn to the skillet, and cook and stir until hot, about 2 minutes.

4. Stir in black beans, and spoon mixture over the lettuce. Top with salsa and sour cream.

MAKES 1 SERVING

326 calories

Prep: 5 minutes

Cook: 10 minutes

You'll need:
large bowl, skillet, nonstick spray

Entire recipe:
326 calories
5.5g total fat
(1.5g sat fat)
684mg sodium
33g carbs
8g fiber
11g sugars
34g protein

Salads & Slaws: Poultry

Chicken Sausage & Apple Salad

The combination of chicken sausage and fruit is amazing. BTW, this salad's delicious with my Honey Mustard Dressing on page 266!

Prep: 5 minutes

Cook: 10 minutes

You'll need:
large bowl, skillet, nonstick spray

Entire recipe:
280 calories
8g total fat
(2.5g sat fat)
678mg sodium
33.5g carbs
7.5g fiber
18.5g sugars
19g protein

3 cups chopped lettuce
3 ounces (about 1 link) fully cooked chicken sausage, sliced into coins
1 cup sliced Fuji or Gala apple
1 cup sliced onion
1 teaspoon chopped garlic
⅛ teaspoon dried thyme
1½ teaspoons Dijon mustard

1. Place lettuce in a large bowl.

2. Bring a skillet sprayed with nonstick spray to medium-high heat. Add sausage, apple, onion, garlic, and thyme. Cook and stir until sausage has browned and onion has softened, about 6 minutes.

3. Stir in mustard, and spoon sausage mixture over the lettuce.

MAKES 1 SERVING

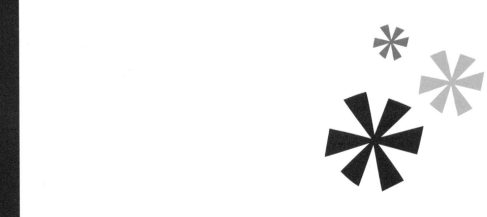

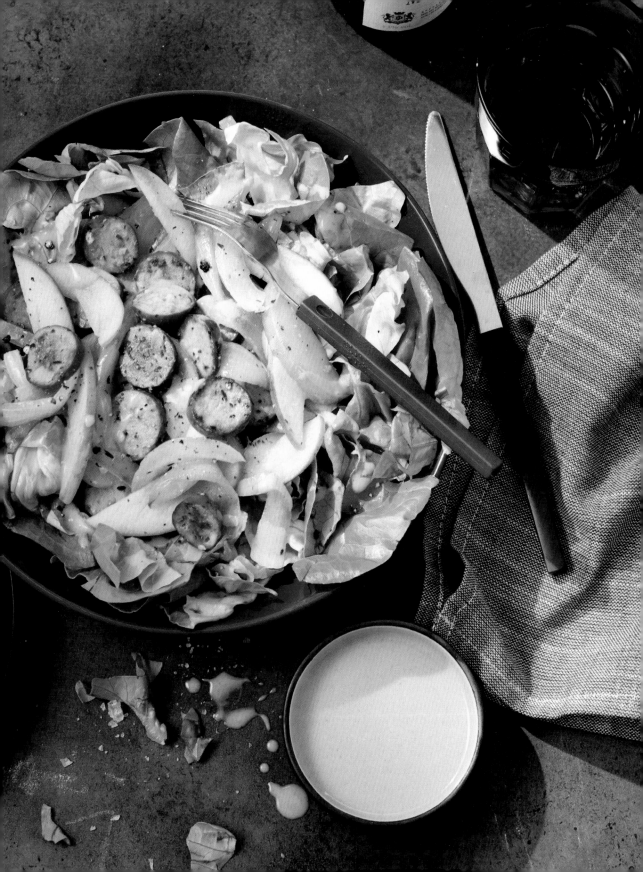

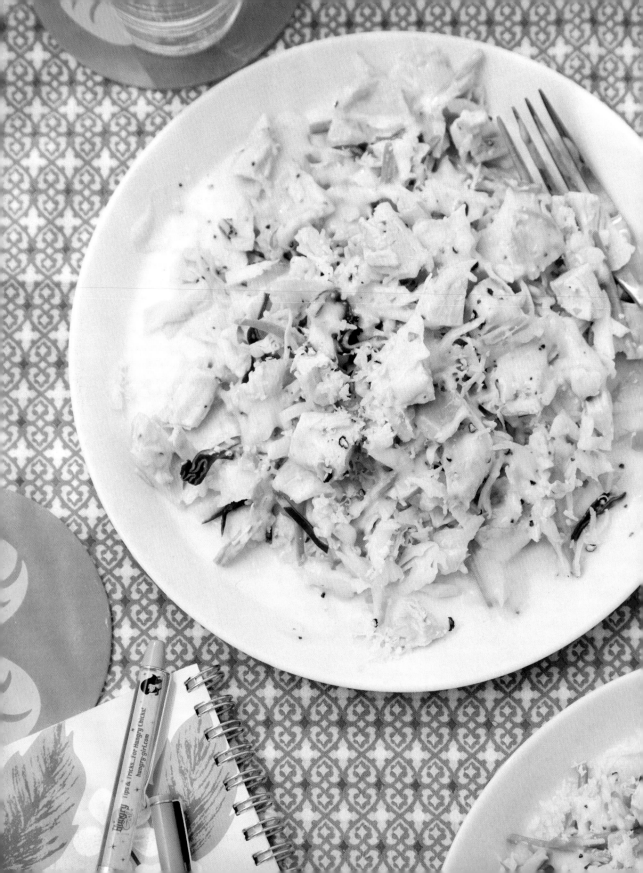

3 cups bagged coleslaw mix
6 ounces cooked skinless chicken breast, cut into
    bite-size pieces
⅓ cup light Caesar dressing
1 tablespoon grated Parmesan cheese

1. Place coleslaw mix and chicken in a large bowl.

2. Add dressing, and toss to coat.

3. Serve topped with Parm.

MAKES 2 SERVINGS

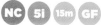

NC **5i** **15m** **GF**

261 calories

Prep: 5 minutes

You'll need:
large bowl

½ of recipe:
261 calories
11.5g total fat
(2.5g sat fat)
482mg sodium
8g carbs
2g fiber
4.5g sugars
29.5g protein

HG Tip
Swap out the chicken for ready-to-eat shrimp, and you've got another 5-minute meal!

Salads & Slaws: Poultry

Blueberries and blackened corn? Who knew?! Prepare for a flavor explosion . . .

3 cups spinach
⅓ cup frozen sweet corn kernels
Dash chili powder
Dash ground cumin
3 ounces cooked skinless chicken breast, cut into bite-size pieces
2 teaspoons lime juice
Dash each salt and black pepper
¼ cup blueberries
2 tablespoons crumbled feta cheese
1 tablespoon chopped fresh cilantro

1. Place spinach in a large bowl.

2. Bring a skillet sprayed with nonstick spray to medium-high heat. Add corn, chili powder, and cumin. Cook and stir until thawed and blackened, about 3 minutes.

3. Add chicken, lime juice, salt, and pepper to the skillet. Cook and stir until hot, about 1 minute.

4. Spoon chicken mixture over the lettuce. Top with blueberries, feta, and cilantro.

MAKES 1 SERVING

Prep: 5 minutes

Cook: 5 minutes

You'll need:
large bowl, skillet, nonstick spray

Entire recipe:
264 calories
6g total fat
(2.5g sat fat)
474mg sodium
19.5g carbs
3.5g fiber
6.5g sugars
32g protein

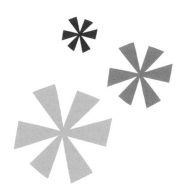

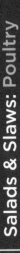
Salads & Slaws: Poultry

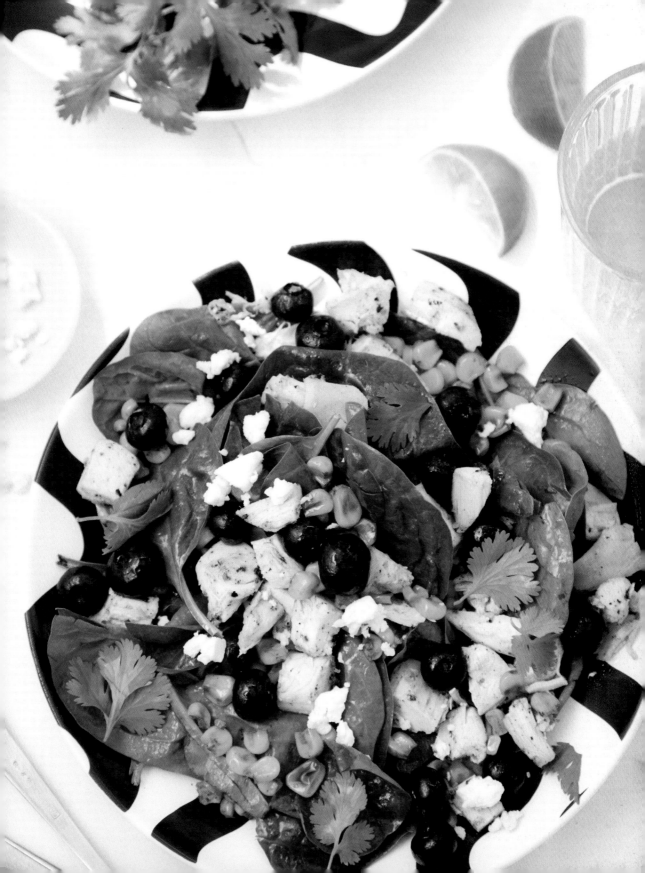

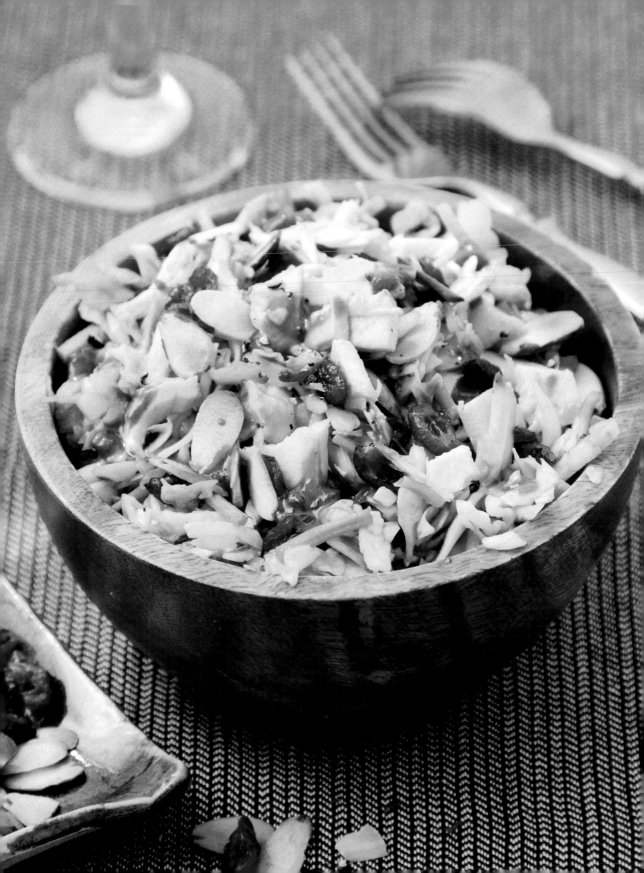

I always keep deli turkey on hand for easy meals like this. It's also great for snacking!

Prep: 10 minutes

You'll need:
large bowl, small bowl

½ of recipe:
235 calories
6g total fat
(0.5g sat fat)
503mg sodium
29g carbs
4g fiber
21g sugars
15g protein

235 calories

4 cups bagged coleslaw mix

4 ounces (about 8 slices) reduced-sodium skinless turkey breast, chopped

¼ cup dried sweetened cranberries, chopped

½ ounce (about 2 tablespoons) sliced almonds

2 tablespoons jellied cranberry sauce

1 tablespoon light mayonnaise

1 teaspoon honey mustard

1 tablespoon balsamic vinegar

Dash each salt and black pepper

1. In a large bowl, combine coleslaw mix, turkey, cranberries, and almonds. Toss to mix.

2. In a small bowl, combine cranberry sauce, mayo, and honey mustard. Stir until smooth. Add vinegar, salt, pepper, and 1 tablespoon water. Mix until uniform.

3. Add cranberry sauce mixture to the large bowl, and toss to coat.

MAKES 2 SERVINGS

HG Tip
Make more of the sauce than the recipe calls for. Then use it as a salad dressing, veggie dip, or flavorful protein topper!

Salads & Slaws: Poultry

Chicken Waldorf Slaw

165 calories

There are so many delicious ways to enjoy this one ... Try it in a whole-wheat pita, in lettuce cups, or over a fresh, crisp salad!

Prep: 10 minutes

You'll need:
large bowl, small bowl

¼th of recipe (about 1 cup):
165 calories
6g total fat
(0.5g sat fat)
386mg sodium
11g carbs
1.5g fiber
7.5g sugars
16g protein

10 ounces canned chicken breast in water, drained and flaked
3 cups bagged coleslaw mix
½ cup chopped Fuji or Gala apple
½ cup seedless grapes, halved
¼ cup finely chopped celery
½ ounce (about 2 tablespoons) chopped walnuts
½ cup fat-free plain Greek yogurt
2 tablespoons light mayonnaise
2 teaspoons Dijon mustard
1 teaspoon lemon juice

1. In a large bowl, combine chicken, coleslaw mix, apple, grapes, celery, and walnuts. Toss to mix.

2. In a small bowl, combine yogurt, mayo, mustard, and lemon juice. Mix until uniform.

3. Add yogurt mixture to the large bowl, and toss to coat.

MAKES 4 SERVINGS

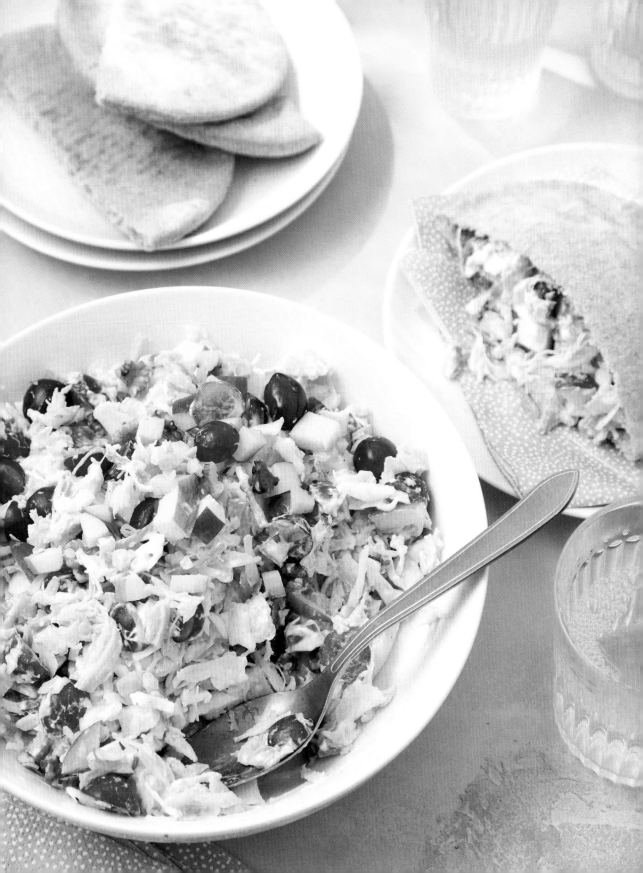

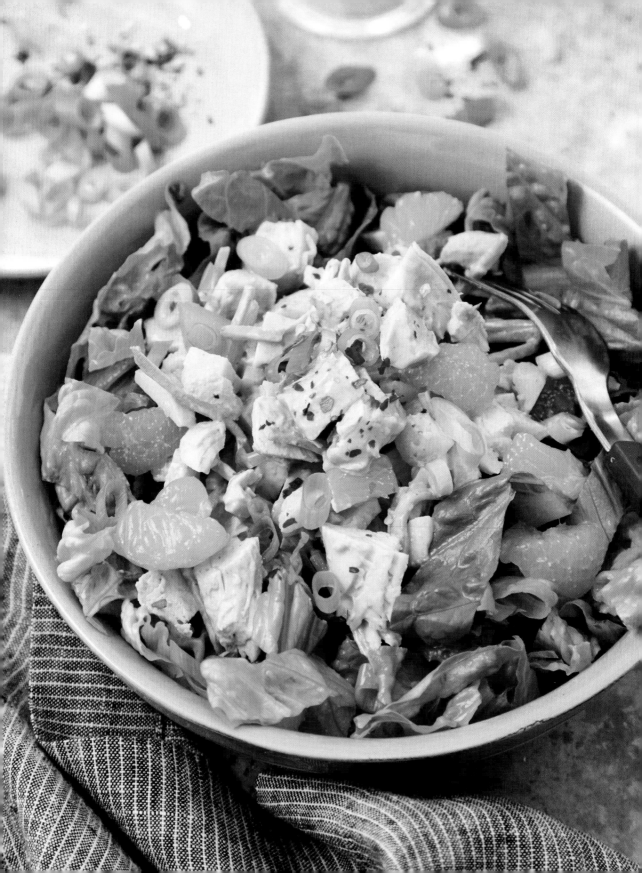

3 cups chopped lettuce

2 tablespoons fat-free plain Greek yogurt

2 tablespoons Thai peanut sauce/salad dressing with 65 calories or less per 2-tablespoon serving

Dash each salt and black pepper

3 ounces cooked skinless chicken breast, cut into bite-size pieces

¼ cup shredded carrots, roughly chopped

¼ cup canned water chestnuts, drained and roughly chopped

2 tablespoons canned mandarin orange segments packed in juice, drained and chopped

2 tablespoons chopped scallions

1. Place lettuce in a large bowl.

2. In a medium bowl, combine yogurt, peanut sauce/ dressing, salt, and pepper. Mix until uniform. Add chicken, carrots, and water chestnuts. Toss to coat.

3. Spoon chicken mixture over the lettuce, and top with oranges and scallions.

MAKES 1 SERVING

NC **15m**

286 calories

Prep: 10 minutes

You'll need:
large bowl,
medium bowl

Entire recipe:
286 calories
6.5g total fat
(1g sat fat)
579mg sodium
24g carbs
5g fiber
13.5g sugars
33g protein

HG Tip
Find peanut sauce at the market near the shelf-stable Asian ingredients. Or whip up my simple Asian-Style Peanut Dressing on page 265!

Salads & Slaws: Poultry

323 calories

3 cups chopped lettuce
1 cup sliced mushrooms
½ cup sliced onion
1½ teaspoons chopped garlic
3 ounces (about 4) raw large shrimp, peeled, tails removed, deveined
3 ounces thinly sliced raw lean flank steak
⅛ teaspoon each salt and black pepper
1 tablespoon sherry cooking wine
2 teaspoons whipped butter

Prep: 10 minutes

Cook: 10 minutes

You'll need:
large bowl, skillet, nonstick spray

Entire recipe:
323 calories
11g total fat
(5g sat fat)
734mg sodium
15.5g carbs
5g fiber
5.5g sugars
40.5g protein

1. Place lettuce in a large bowl.

2. Bring a skillet sprayed with nonstick spray to medium-high heat. Add mushrooms, onion, and garlic. Cook and stir until slightly softened, about 3 minutes.

3. Add shrimp, steak, salt, and pepper. Cook and stir until veggies have softened and shrimp and steak are fully cooked, about 3 more minutes.

4. Add sherry and butter. Cook and stir until melted and mixed, about 1 minute.

5. Spoon mixture over the lettuce.

MAKES 1 SERVING

HG Tip
Pop the steak in the freezer for 10 minutes before preparing this recipe . . . This makes it easier to thinly slice!

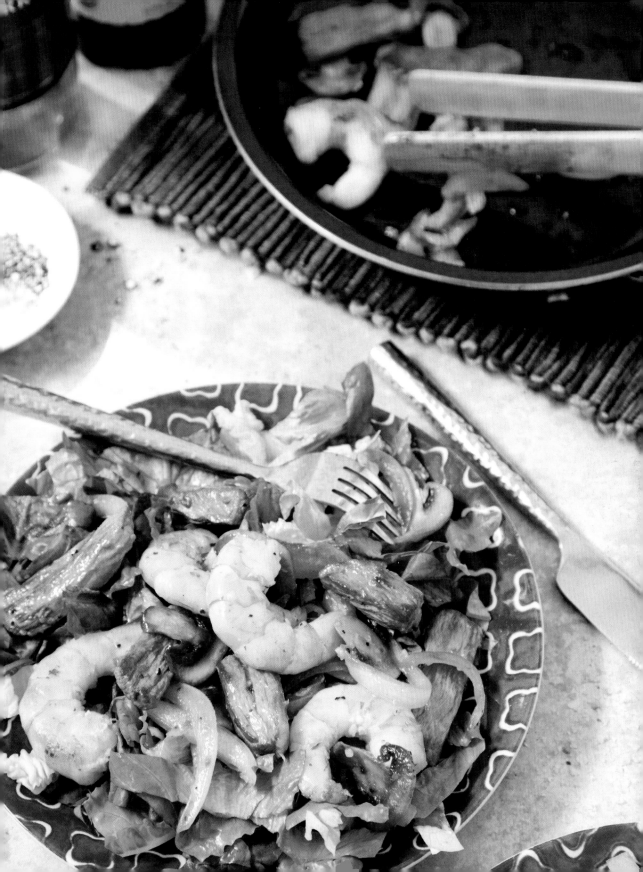

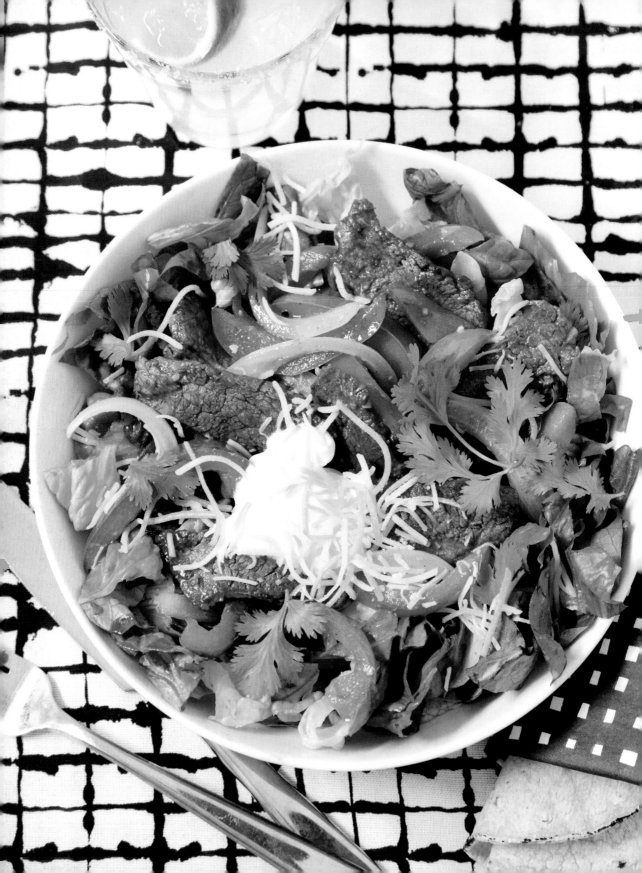

Steak Fajita Salad

3 cups chopped lettuce
½ cup sliced bell pepper
½ cup sliced onion
4 ounces thinly sliced raw lean flank steak
2 teaspoons fajita seasoning
2 teaspoons chopped garlic
1 teaspoon lime juice
2 tablespoons shredded reduced-fat Mexican-blend cheese
2 tablespoons light sour cream
1 tablespoon chopped fresh cilantro

1. Place lettuce in a large bowl.

2. Bring a skillet sprayed with nonstick spray to medium-high heat. Add pepper and onion. Cook and stir until slightly softened and lightly browned, about 5 minutes.

3. Add steak, fajita seasoning, garlic, and lime juice. Cook and stir until veggies have softened and steak is fully cooked, about 3 minutes.

4. Spoon steak mixture over the lettuce, and top with cheese, sour cream, and cilantro.

MAKES 1 SERVING

Prep: 10 minutes

Cook: 10 minutes

You'll need:
large bowl, skillet, nonstick spray

Entire recipe:
330 calories
13g total fat
(6g sat fat)
570mg sodium
20.5g carbs
5g fiber
8.5g sugars
32.5g protein

330 calories

Salads & Slaws: Beef & Pork

Steakhouse Spinach Salad

308 calories

15m GF

Romaine is my usual go-to for salad greens, but it's nice to change things up! Spinach pairs perfectly with the steak and blue cheese.

Prep: 10 minutes

Cook: 5 minutes

You'll need:
large bowl, skillet, nonstick spray

Entire recipe:
308 calories
13g total fat
(6.5g sat fat)
698mg sodium
12.5g carbs
4g fiber
5.5g sugars
34.5 protein

3 cups spinach
½ cup chopped tomatoes
4 ounces thinly sliced raw lean flank steak
⅓ cup chopped onion
Dash each salt and black pepper
2 tablespoons crumbled blue cheese
1 tablespoon precooked crumbled bacon

1. Place spinach in a large bowl. Top with tomatoes.

2. Bring a skillet sprayed with nonstick spray to medium-high heat. Add steak, onion, salt, and pepper. Cook and stir until steak is fully cooked and onion has softened, about 3 minutes.

3. Spoon steak mixture over the salad, and top with blue cheese and bacon.

MAKES 1 SERVING

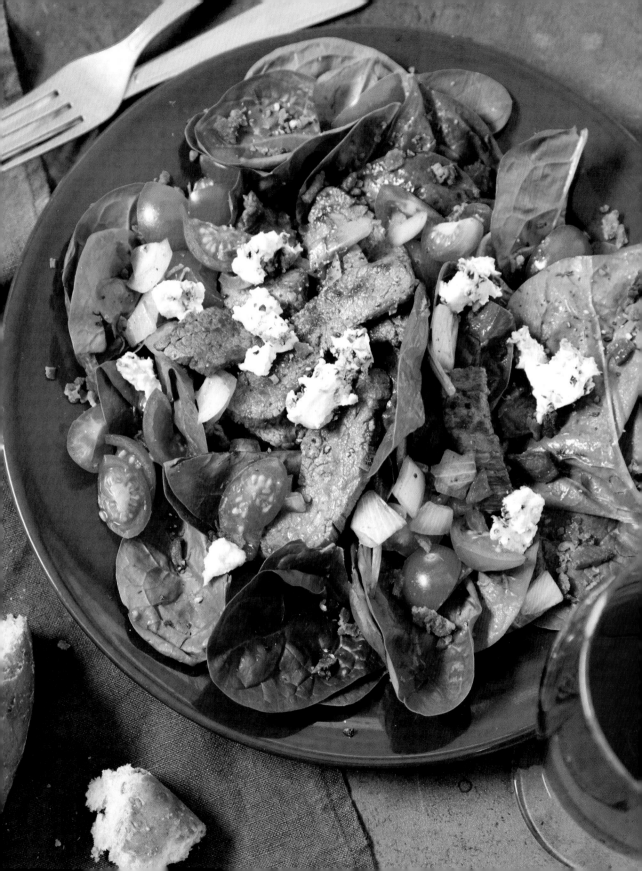

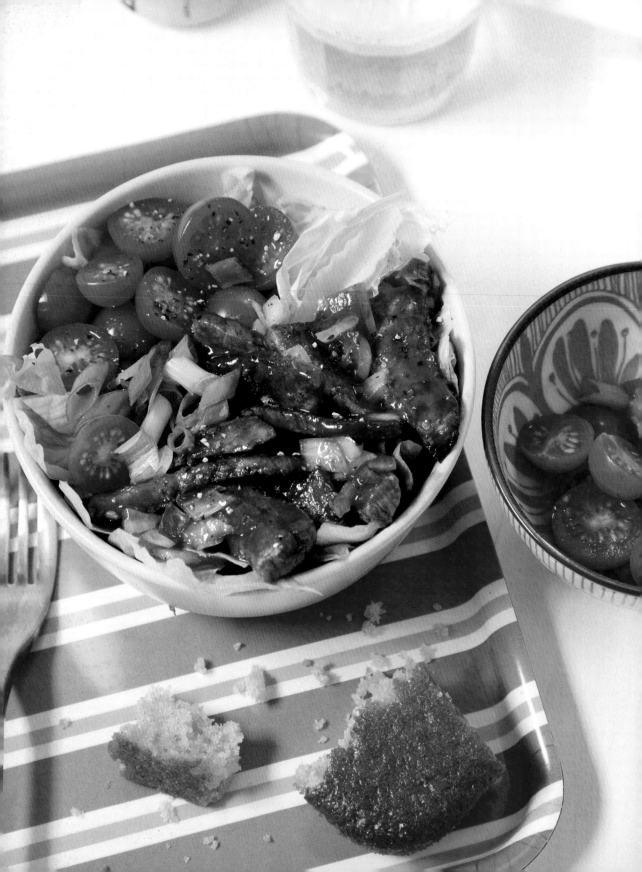

Honey BBQ Steak Salad

Salad dressing suggestion! Grab a light honey mustard for this one, or whip up my recipe on page 266.

Prep: 5 minutes

Cook: 5 minutes

You'll need:
large bowl, small bowl, skillet, nonstick spray

Entire recipe:
336 calories
7.5g total fat
(3g sat fat)
588mg sodium
40g carbs
4.5g fiber
30.5g sugars
27.5g protein

336 calories

3 cups chopped lettuce
½ cup cherry tomatoes, halved
2 tablespoons BBQ sauce with about 45 calories per 2-tablespoon serving
1 tablespoon honey
4 ounces thinly sliced raw lean flank steak
¼ cup chopped red onion
⅛ teaspoon garlic powder
⅛ teaspoon onion powder
Dash each salt and black pepper
1 tablespoon chopped scallions

1. Place lettuce in a large bowl. Top with tomatoes.

2. In a small bowl, mix BBQ sauce with honey until uniform.

3. Bring a skillet sprayed with nonstick spray to medium-high heat. Add steak, onion, and seasonings. Cook and stir until steak is fully cooked and onion has softened, about 3 minutes.

4. Remove skillet from heat. Add honey BBQ sauce, and mix well.

5. Spoon steak mixture over the salad, and top with scallions.

MAKES 1 SERVING

Mediterranean Tuna Slaw

209 calories

3 cups bagged broccoli slaw
5 ounces albacore tuna packed in water, drained and flaked
½ cup cherry tomatoes, halved
¼ cup finely chopped red onion
¼ cup sliced Kalamata olives
¼ cup light Italian dressing
½ teaspoon dried oregano
2 tablespoons crumbled feta cheese

1. In a large bowl, combine broccoli slaw, tuna, tomatoes, onion, and olives. Add dressing and oregano, and toss to coat.

2. Serve topped with feta.

MAKES 2 SERVINGS

Prep: 10 minutes

You'll need:
large bowl

½ of recipe
(about 2 cups):
209 calories
9g total fat
(2g sat fat)
791mg sodium
15.5g carbs
5g fiber
7g sugars
17g protein

HG FYI

Chilling is optional, but the longer this dish chills, the more flavorful it becomes. Great for make-ahead meals!

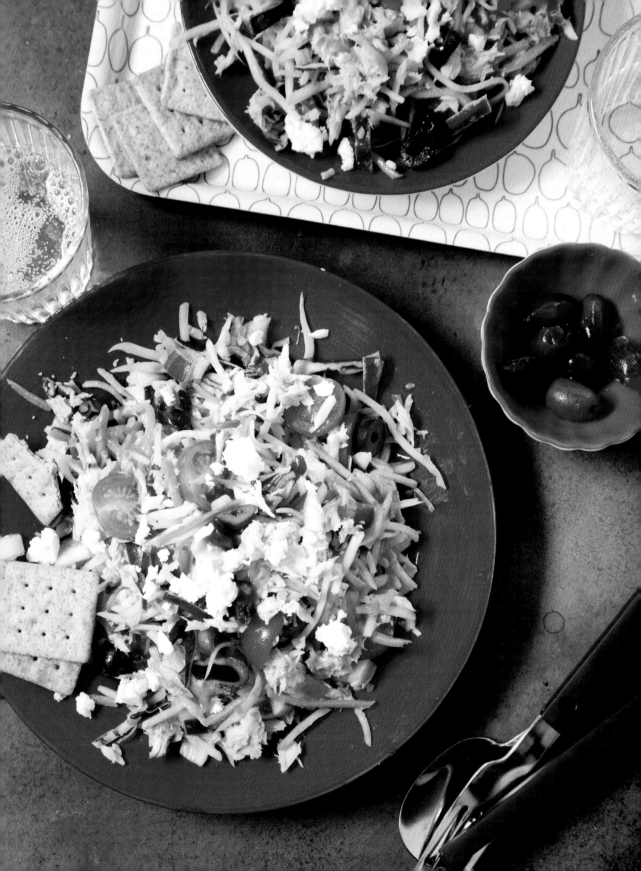

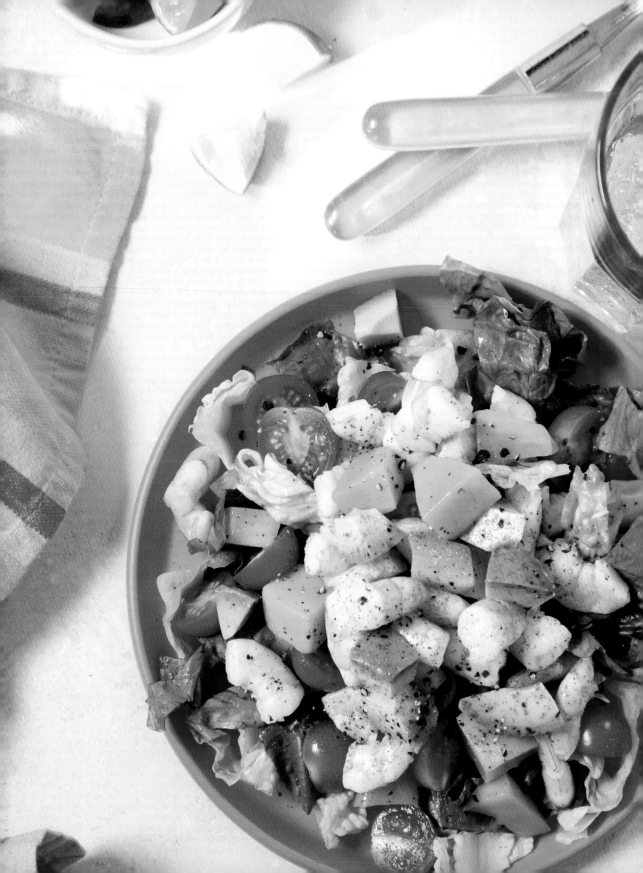

Shrimp & Mango Salad

Salads like this are why I almost always have shrimp in my freezer. And mango makes everything better . . .

3 cups chopped lettuce
½ cup cherry tomatoes, halved
3 ounces (about 6 large) ready-to-eat shrimp, chopped
2 ounces (about ¼ cup) chopped avocado
¼ cup chopped mango
2 teaspoons lime juice
Dash Cajun seasoning
Dash ground cumin
Dash salt

1. Place lettuce in a large bowl. Top with tomatoes.

2. In a medium bowl, combine remaining ingredients, and toss to coat.

3. Spoon shrimp mixture over the salad.

MAKES 1 SERVING

NC **15m** **GF**

253 calories

Prep: 10 minutes

You'll need:
large bowl,
medium bowl

Entire recipe:
253 calories
10g total fat
(1.5g sat fat)
389mg sodium
21g carbs
8.5g fiber
10.5g sugars
23.5g protein

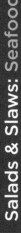

Pssst . . .
Don't forget about all the DIY salad dressings, starting on page 263!

Salads & Slaws: Seafood

Seafood Sunomono Salad

This one's inspired by the yummy cucumber salads at sushi restaurants. Just a little bit of sesame oil adds BIG-TIME flavor.

Prep: 5 minutes

Chill: 15 minutes

You'll need:
large bowl

Entire recipe:
213 calories
7.5g total fat
(1g sat fat)
828mg sodium
15.5g carbs
2.5g fiber
12g sugars
21g protein

1½ tablespoons seasoned rice vinegar, or more to taste
1 teaspoon sesame oil
1 large cucumber, halved lengthwise, seeded, and thinly sliced
1½ ounces ready-to-eat bay shrimp
1½ ounces canned lump crabmeat, drained
1 teaspoon sesame seeds

1. In a large bowl, mix vinegar with oil. Add cucumber, shrimp, and crab. Toss to mix.

2. Cover and refrigerate for at least 15 minutes.

3. Top with sesame seeds.

MAKES 1 SERVING

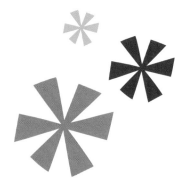

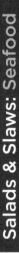

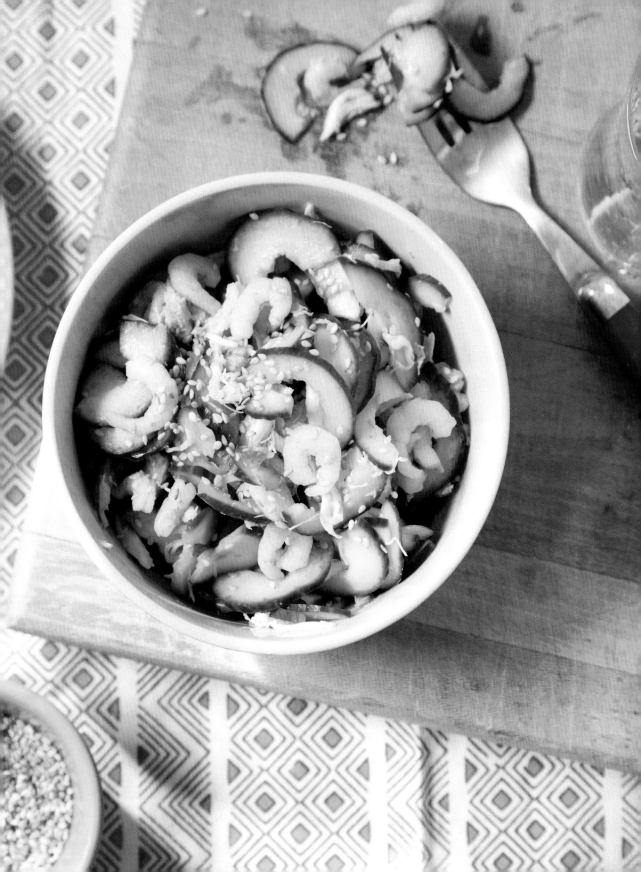

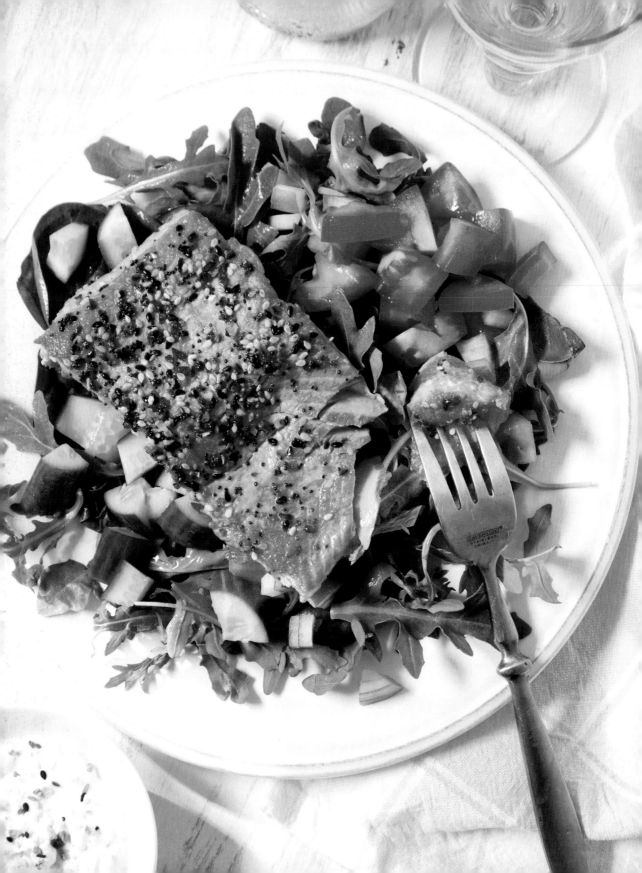

Everything Bagel Salmon Salad

Everything bagel seasoning is seriously magical. I created the Everything Bagel Dressing on page 266 with this recipe in mind!

One 4-ounce raw skinless salmon fillet
½ teaspoon everything bagel seasoning, or more for topping
3 cups chopped lettuce
½ cup chopped cucumber
⅓ cup chopped tomato
1 tablespoon finely chopped red onion

1. Preheat oven to 450 degrees. Spray a baking sheet with nonstick spray.

2. Place salmon on the baking sheet, and sprinkle with bagel seasoning. Bake until cooked through, about 14 minutes.

3. Meanwhile, place lettuce in a large bowl. Top with cucumber, tomato, and onion.

4. Top salad with salmon.

MAKES 1 SERVING

  GF

239 calories

Prep: 5 minutes

Cook: 15 minutes

You'll need:
baking sheet,
nonstick spray,
large bowl

Entire recipe:
239 calories
9.5g total fat
(2.5g sat fat)
253mg sodium
10g carbs
4g fiber
4.5g sugars
26g protein

Salads & Slaws: Seafood

Smoked Salmon Citrus Salad

3 cups arugula

½ cup grapefruit segments packed in juice, drained

2½ ounces roughly chopped smoked salmon with 300mg sodium or less per ounce

2 ounces (about ½ cup) sliced avocado

1 tablespoon chopped fresh dill

1. Place arugula in a large bowl.

2. Top with grapefruit, salmon, avocado, and dill.

MAKES 1 SERVING

Prep: 5 minutes

You'll need:
large bowl

Entire recipe:
233 calories
11.5g total fat
(2g sat fat)
779mg sodium
18.5g carbs
5.5g fiber
12.5g sugars
16.5g protein

HG Tip
If you can't find grapefruit packed in juice, go for the kind packed in light syrup and give it a quick rinse . . .

Salads & Slaws: Seafood

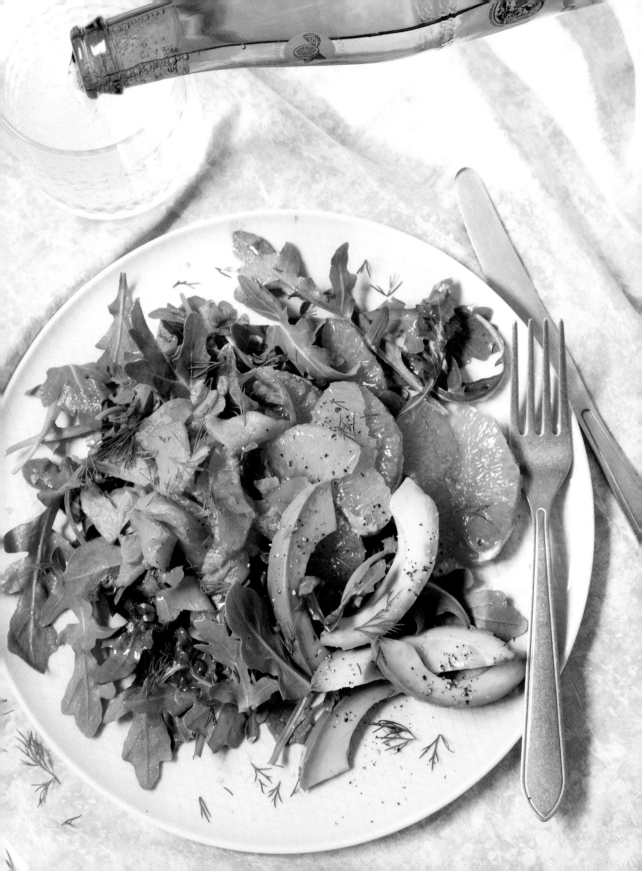

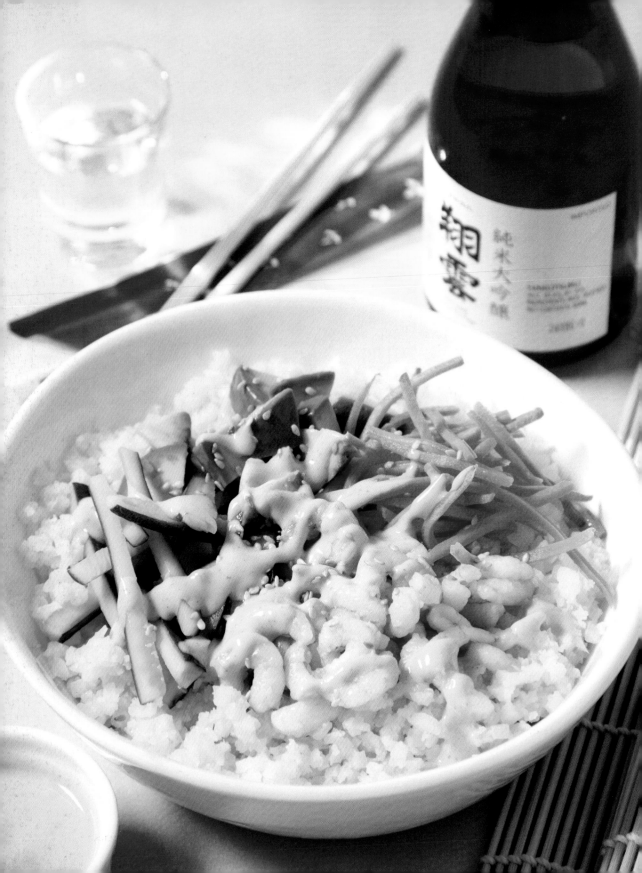

Spicy Shrimp Sushi Roll in a Bowl

More sushi-inspired deliciousness! And if you're not a fan of spicy food, just leave out the sriracha.

1½ cups frozen riced cauliflower
1½ teaspoons seasoned rice vinegar, or more to taste
3 ounces ready-to-eat bay shrimp
1 ounce (about 2 tablespoons) chopped avocado
⅓ cup shredded carrots
⅓ cup seedless cucumber cut into matchstick-size strips
½ teaspoon sesame seeds
1 tablespoon light mayonnaise
1 teaspoon sriracha hot chili sauce
Optional topping: soy sauce

1. Place cauliflower in a medium microwave-safe bowl. Cover and microwave for 2 minutes, or until thawed and warm.

2. Stir in vinegar. Let cool for 15 minutes.

3. Top with shrimp, avocado, carrots, cucumber, and sesame seeds.

4. In a small bowl, combine mayo, chili sauce, and 1 teaspoon water. Stir until uniform, and drizzle over the bowl.

MAKES 1 SERVING

Prep: 10 minutes
Cook: 5 minutes
Cool: 15 minutes

You'll need:
medium microwave-safe bowl, small bowl

Entire recipe:
275 calories
10.5g total fat
(1.5g sat fat)
738mg sodium
21.5g carbs
7.5g fiber
10g sugars
25.5g protein

275 calories

HG Tip
No bay shrimp? Just chop up some large shrimp.

Salads & Slaws: Seafood

Honey Mustard Tuna Salad

293 calories

Add honey mustard to tuna salad for a flavor explosion! Try the tuna part of this recipe in sandwiches and wraps too.

Prep: 10 minutes

You'll need:
large bowl,
medium bowl

Entire recipe:
293 calories
9g total fat
(1g sat fat)
644mg sodium
22g carbs
5.5g fiber
12g sugars
30g protein

3 cups chopped lettuce
5 ounces albacore tuna packed in water, drained and flaked
1½ tablespoons fat-free plain Greek yogurt
1½ tablespoons light mayonnaise
2 teaspoons honey mustard
1 teaspoon sweet relish
¼ cup finely chopped bell pepper
¼ cup finely chopped carrot
¼ cup finely chopped red onion
Optional topping: chopped fresh dill

1. Place lettuce in a large bowl.

2. In a medium bowl, combine tuna, yogurt, mayo, honey mustard, and relish. Mix until uniform.

3. Stir in pepper, carrot, and onion, and spoon tuna mixture over the lettuce.

MAKES 1 SERVING

Salads & Slaws: Seafood

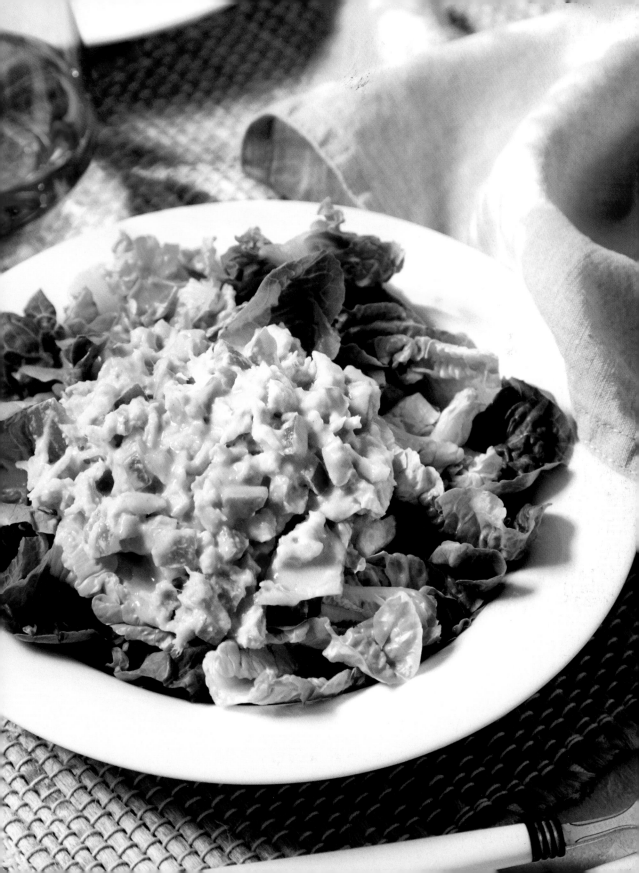

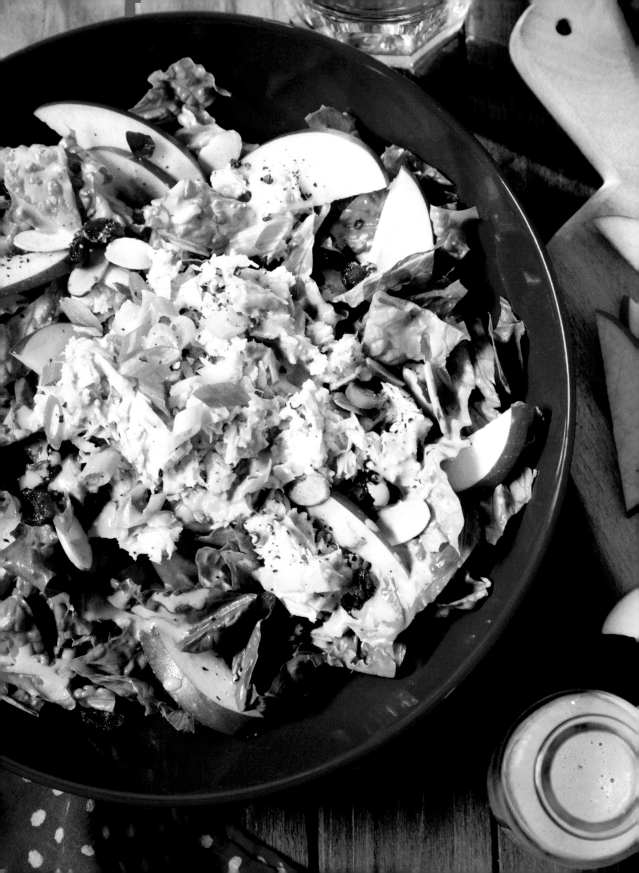

This one's delicious with a light balsamic vinaigrette ... and I just happen to have a recipe for a creamy one on page 264!

Prep: 5 minutes

You'll need:
large bowl

272 calories

Entire recipe:
272 calories
6.5g total fat
(0.5g sat fat)
466mg sodium
27.5g carbs
6.5g fiber
18.5g sugars
28.5g protein

3 cups chopped lettuce
½ cup sliced Fuji or Gala apple
2 tablespoons sweetened dried cranberries, chopped
5 ounces albacore tuna packed in water, drained and flaked
Dash each salt and black pepper
2 tablespoons chopped scallions
¼ ounce (about 1 tablespoon) sliced almonds

1. Place lettuce in a large bowl. Top with apple and cranberries.

2. Add tuna, and sprinkle with salt and pepper. Top with scallions and almonds.

MAKES 1 SERVING

Salads & Slaws: Seafood

Succotash Salad

300 calories

2 cups finely chopped lettuce
⅓ cup frozen sweet corn kernels
⅓ cup frozen shelled edamame
1 tablespoon olive oil
⅓ cup finely chopped asparagus
⅓ cup finely chopped zucchini
2 tablespoons vegetable broth
½ cup chopped and seeded tomato
¼ cup finely chopped jicama
1 teaspoon lime juice
⅛ teaspoon salt
Dash black pepper
2 tablespoons chopped fresh cilantro

1. Place lettuce in a large bowl.

2. Bring a skillet sprayed with nonstick spray to medium-high heat. Add corn, edamame, and oil. Cook and stir until lightly browned, about 3 minutes.

3. Add asparagus, zucchini, and broth. Cover and cook for 3 minutes, or until softened.

4. Reduce heat to medium low. Add tomato and jicama. Cook and stir until hot and well mixed, about 1 minute.

5. Remove skillet from heat. Mix in lime juice, salt, and pepper.

6. Spoon mixture over lettuce. Serve topped with cilantro.

MAKES 1 SERVING

Prep: 10 minutes

Cook: 10 minutes

You'll need:
large bowl, skillet with lid, nonstick spray

Entire recipe:
300 calories
17g total fat
(2g sat fat)
412mg sodium
29g carbs
9.5g fiber
9.5g sugars
11g protein

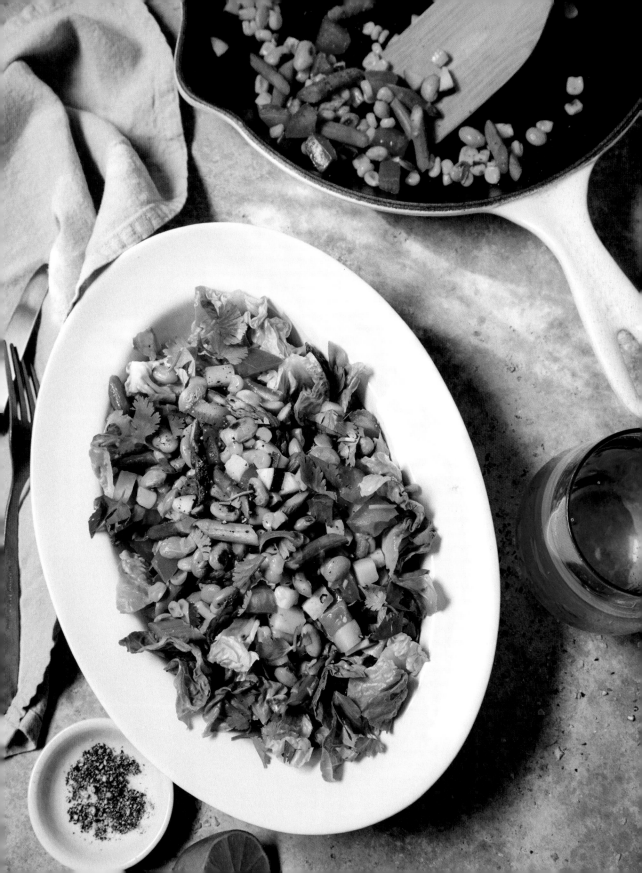

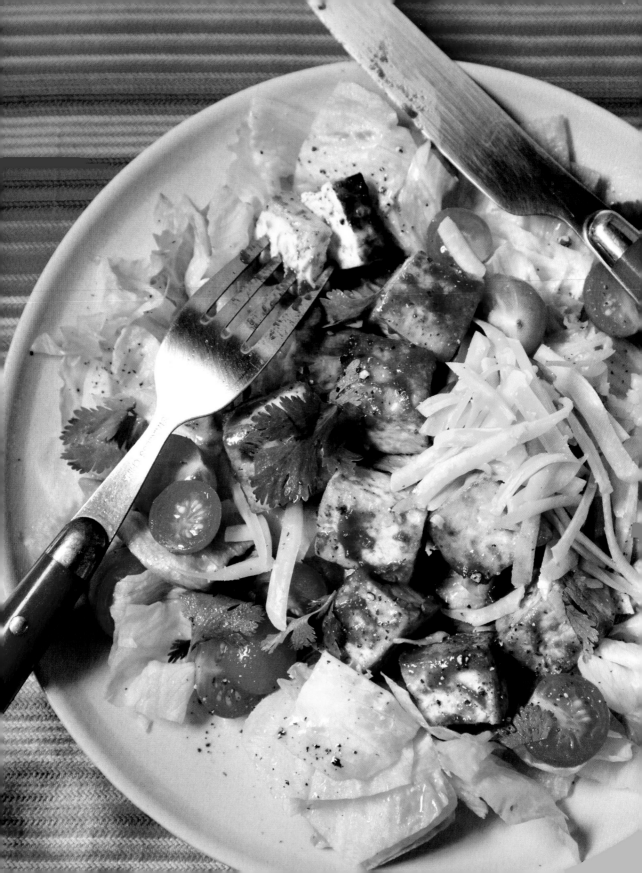

BBQ Tofu Salad

3 cups chopped lettuce

4 ounces block-style extra-firm tofu, excess moisture removed, cut into 1-inch cubes

¼ teaspoon garlic powder

Dash salt

2 tablespoons BBQ sauce with 45 calories or less per 2-tablespoon serving

½ cup cherry tomatoes, halved

¼ cup shredded reduced-fat cheddar cheese

1 tablespoon chopped fresh cilantro

1. Place lettuce in a large bowl.

2. Bring a skillet sprayed with nonstick spray to medium-high heat. Add tofu, garlic powder, and salt. Cook until golden brown, about 10 minutes, gently flipping to brown on all sides.

3. Transfer tofu to a medium bowl. Add BBQ sauce, and gently toss to coat.

4. Spoon BBQ tofu over the lettuce, and top with tomatoes, cheese, and cilantro.

MAKES 1 SERVING

15m V GF

290 calories

Prep: 5 minutes

Cook: 10 minutes

You'll need:
large bowl, skillet, nonstick spray, medium bowl

Entire recipe:
290 calories
13g total fat
(4.5g sat fat)
739mg sodium
21.5g carbs
4.5g fiber
12g sugars
22.5g protein

HG Tip

Use paper towels to remove as much moisture as possible from the tofu before cooking. It'll crisp up way better!

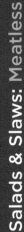

Salads & Slaws: Meatless

Berries & Feta Kale Salad

I'm not typically a fan of raw kale, but this salad's fantastic. That massage tip below really makes a big difference!

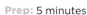

Prep: 5 minutes

You'll need:
large bowl

Entire recipe:
268 calories
13g total fat
(5g sat fat)
526mg sodium
29g carbs
9.5g fiber
14.5g sugars
12g protein

3 cups chopped kale
2 tablespoons balsamic vinegar
Dash each salt and black pepper
½ cup blackberries
½ cup sliced strawberries
¼ cup crumbled feta cheese
½ ounce (about 2 tablespoons) chopped pistachios

1. Place kale in a large bowl. Add vinegar, salt, and pepper, and toss to coat.

2. Top with blackberries, strawberries, feta, and pistachios.

MAKES 1 SERVING

HG Tip
It might sound funny, but give your kale a massage to make it more tender and less chewy! Just knead the leaves with your hands before adding the vinegar and seasonings.

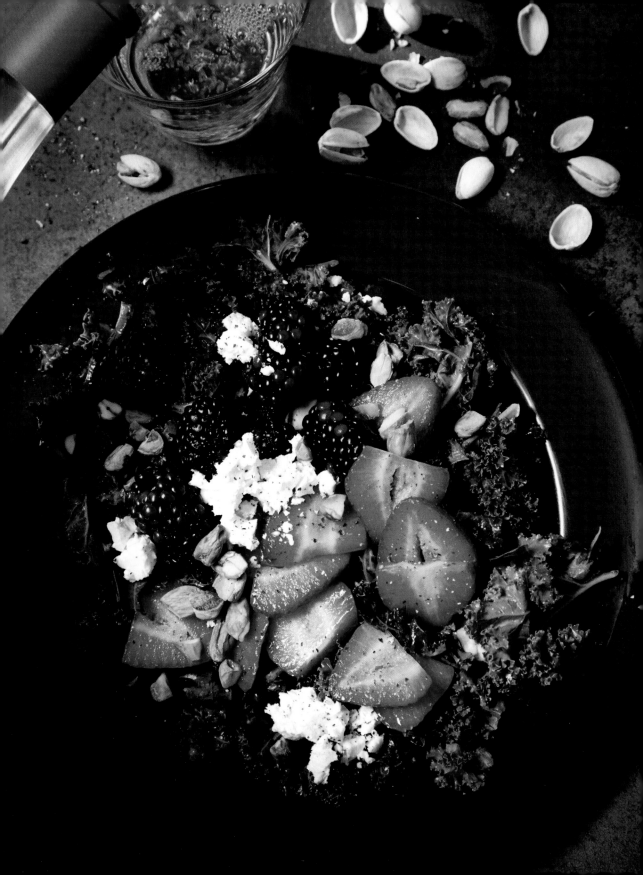

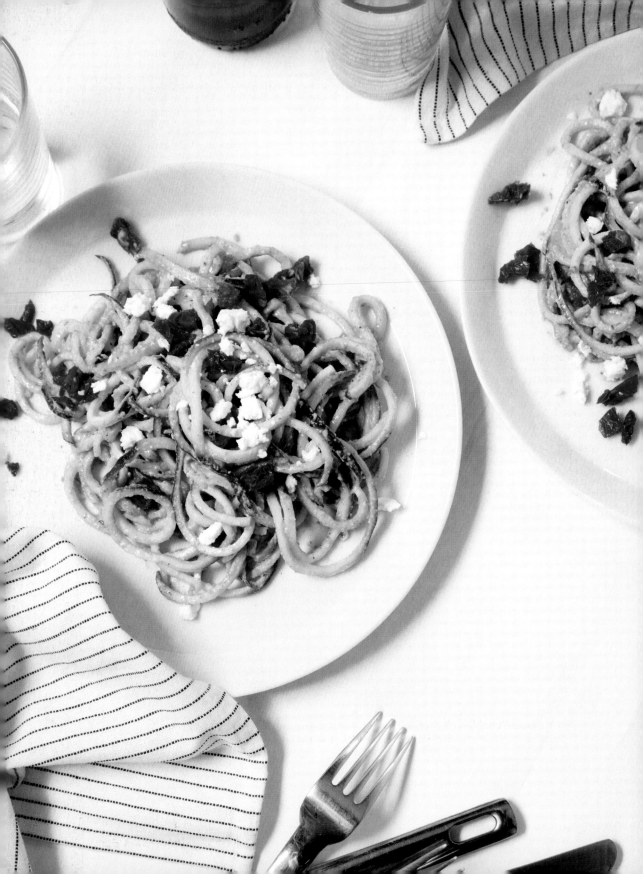

Pesto Zucchini-Noodle Salad

I like to give premade pesto sauce more bang for the calorie buck by making it go further with smart-choice creamy ingredients. Ricotta's the star here!

Prep: 5 minutes

Chill: 15 minutes

You'll need:
small bowl, large bowl

½ the recipe (about 2 cups):
265 calories
18g total fat
(5g sat fat)
606mg sodium
18.5g carbs
4g fiber
11.5g sugars
10.5g protein

265 calories

¼ cup pesto sauce

3 tablespoons light/low-fat ricotta cheese

2 tablespoons light/reduced-fat cream cheese, room temperature

⅛ teaspoon salt

20 ounces (about 2 large) spiralized zucchini, roughly chopped

2 tablespoons chopped bagged sun-dried tomatoes (not packed in oil)

2 tablespoons crumbled feta cheese

1. To make the sauce, in a small bowl, combine pesto, ricotta, cream cheese, and salt. Stir until uniform.

2. Place zucchini noodles in a large bowl. Add sauce, and toss to coat. Cover and refrigerate until chilled, about 15 minutes.

3. Stir well, and serve topped with tomatoes and feta.

MAKES 2 SERVINGS

HG Tip
The nutritional info for pesto sauce can vary widely. When shopping, turn the jars around, and look for the option with the fewest calories and least fat.

Salads & Slaws: Meatless

Mediterranean Lentil Salad

237 calories

The DIY tzatziki swap totally makes this recipe. For a vegan-friendly spin, use a dairy-free yogurt swap.

Prep: 10 minutes

You'll need:
medium bowl, large bowl

Entire recipe:
237 calories
3.5g total fat
(0.5g sat fat)
728mg sodium
37g carbs
11g fiber
10g sugars
17g protein

Yogurt Sauce
¼ cup fat-free plain Greek yogurt
1 teaspoon dried dill
1 teaspoon white wine vinegar
½ teaspoon lemon juice
¼ teaspoon garlic powder
⅛ teaspoon salt

Salad
3 cups chopped lettuce
½ cup chopped cucumber
½ cup cooked ready-to-eat lentils
½ cup chopped tomato
¼ cup chopped red onion
2 tablespoons sliced black or Kalamata olives

1. In a medium bowl, mix sauce ingredients until smooth and uniform.

2. Place lettuce in a large bowl. Top with remaining salad ingredients.

3. Spoon sauce over salad.

MAKES 1 SERVING

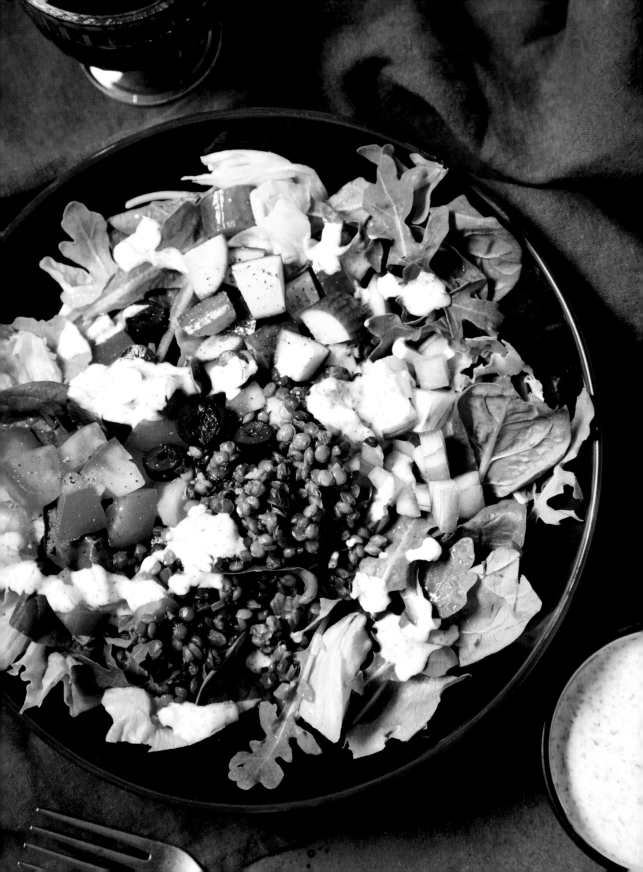

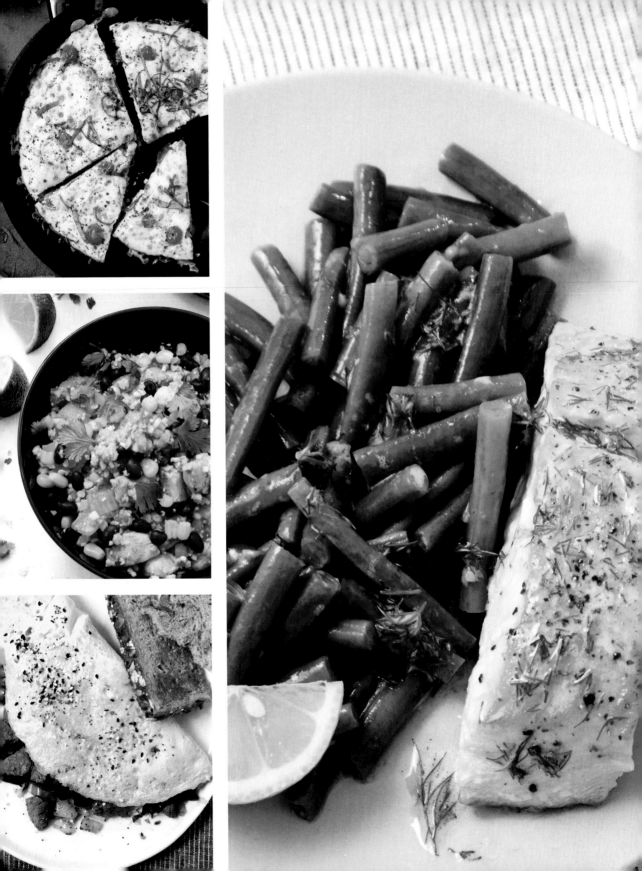

2

Stir-Frys & Skillet Meals

Stir-frying is one of my favorite ways to save time in the kitchen. So quick—and the flavor possibilities are endless. In this chapter, I'm also bringing you meatballs, frittatas . . . even a yummy Mexican pizza!

Chicken Cordon Bleu Stir-Fry

332 calories

So cheesy & comforting. This dish is one of my all-time favorites!

2 tablespoons panko bread crumbs
2 tablespoons grated Parmesan cheese
¼ teaspoon garlic powder
¼ teaspoon onion powder
2 dashes each salt and black pepper
8 ounces raw boneless skinless chicken breast, cut into bite-size pieces
6 cups roughly chopped spinach
1 ounce (about 2 slices) reduced-sodium ham, roughly chopped
2 slices reduced-fat Swiss cheese, broken into pieces
2 tablespoons light/reduced-fat cream cheese
1 tablespoon Dijon mustard

Prep: 5 minutes

Cook: 10 minutes

You'll need:
skillet, nonstick spray

½ of recipe:
332 calories
13g total fat
(6g sat fat)
837mg sodium
9g carbs
2g fiber
2g sugars
42.5g protein

1. Bring a skillet sprayed with nonstick spray to medium heat. Add panko, Parm, ⅛ teaspoon garlic powder, ⅛ teaspoon onion powder, and a dash each salt and pepper. Cook and stir until crispy and browned, about 2 minutes. Set aside for topping.

2. Remove skillet from heat, respray, and bring to medium-high heat. Add chicken and remaining ⅛ teaspoon garlic powder, ⅛ teaspoon onion powder, and dash each salt and pepper. Cook and stir until lightly browned, about 3 minutes.

3. Add spinach and ham, and cook until spinach has wilted, about 2 minutes. Add Swiss, cream cheese, and mustard. Cook and stir until cheeses have melted, sauce is uniform, and chicken is fully cooked, about 1 minute.

4. Serve topped with panko mixture.

MAKES 2 SERVINGS

> ### HG Alternative
> **Avoiding gluten? Use gluten-free panko, or skip the bread crumbs altogether.**

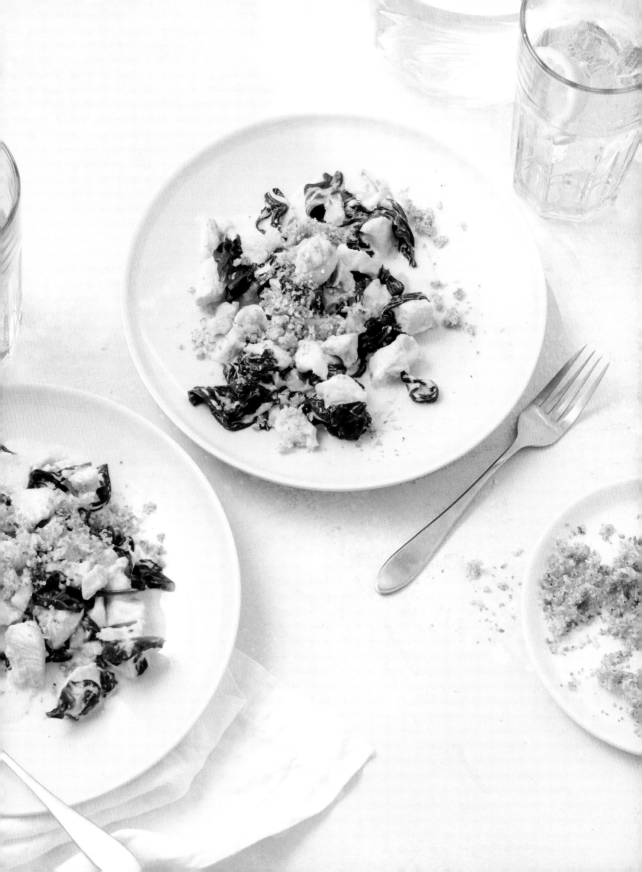

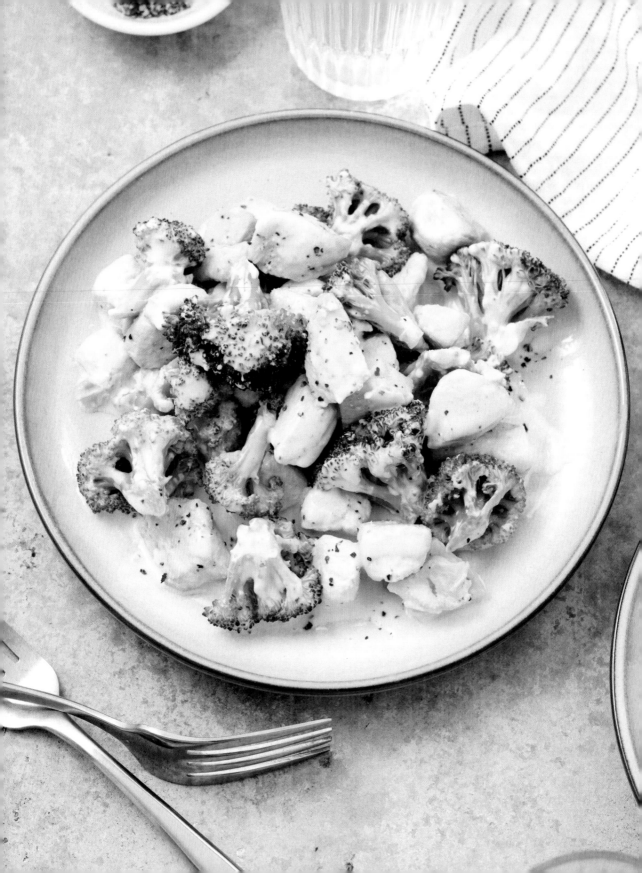

Cheesy Chicken & Broccoli Stir-Fry

It never fails to amaze me how much rich deliciousness cream cheese brings to a dish, and this speedy dinner is no exception!

272 calories

Prep: 5 minutes

Cook: 15 minutes

You'll need:
skillet with lid, nonstick spray

½ of recipe:
272 calories
9g total fat
(4g sat fat)
373mg sodium
12g carbs
4.5g fiber
5.5g sugars
32g protein

4 cups frozen broccoli florets
8 ounces raw boneless skinless chicken breast, cut into
   bite-size pieces
⅛ teaspoon each salt and black pepper
¼ cup light/reduced-fat cream cheese
½ teaspoon garlic powder
½ teaspoon onion powder

1. Bring a skillet sprayed with nonstick spray to medium-high heat. Add frozen broccoli and 2 tablespoons water. Cover and cook for 6 minutes, or until thawed.

2. Add chicken, salt, and pepper. Cook and stir until broccoli is hot and chicken is fully cooked, about 5 minutes.

3. Reduce heat to medium low. Add cream cheese, garlic powder, and onion powder. Cook and stir until melted and well mixed, about 1 minute.

MAKES 2 SERVINGS

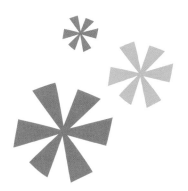

Stir-Frys & Skillet Meals: Poultry

Chicken Sausage Primavera

261 calories

Precooked chicken sausage is perfect for speedy meals like this. And browning it really brings out the flavor!

Prep: 5 minutes

Cook: 15 minutes

You'll need:
microwave-safe bowl, skillet, nonstick spray

½ of recipe:
261 calories
10.5g total fat
(3g sat fat)
854mg sodium
23g carbs
7g fiber
11.5g sugars
20g protein

3 cups bagged broccoli slaw
1 cup sliced bell pepper
1 cup sliced onion
6 ounces (about 2 links) fully cooked chicken sausage, sliced into coins
⅔ cup marinara sauce with 70 calories or less per ½-cup serving
2 teaspoons grated Parmesan cheese

1. Place broccoli slaw in a microwave-safe bowl with ¼ cup water. Cover and microwave for 3 minutes, or until softened.

2. Meanwhile, bring a skillet sprayed with nonstick spray to medium-high heat. Add pepper and onion, and cook until slightly softened and lightly browned, about 3 minutes.

3. Add sausage to the skillet, and cook and stir until browned, about 4 minutes.

4. Add slaw and marinara. Cook and stir until hot and well mixed, about 2 minutes.

5. Serve topped with Parm.

MAKES 2 SERVINGS

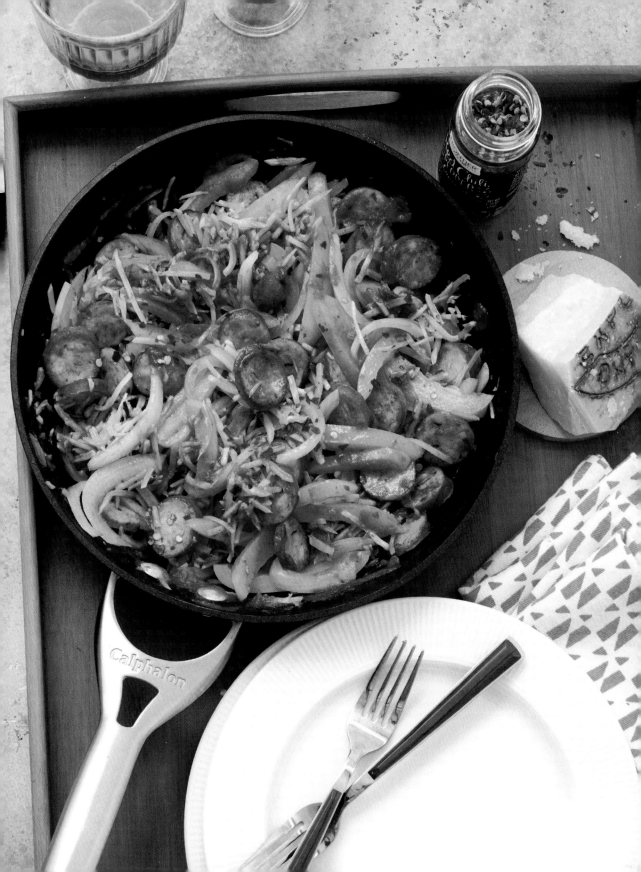

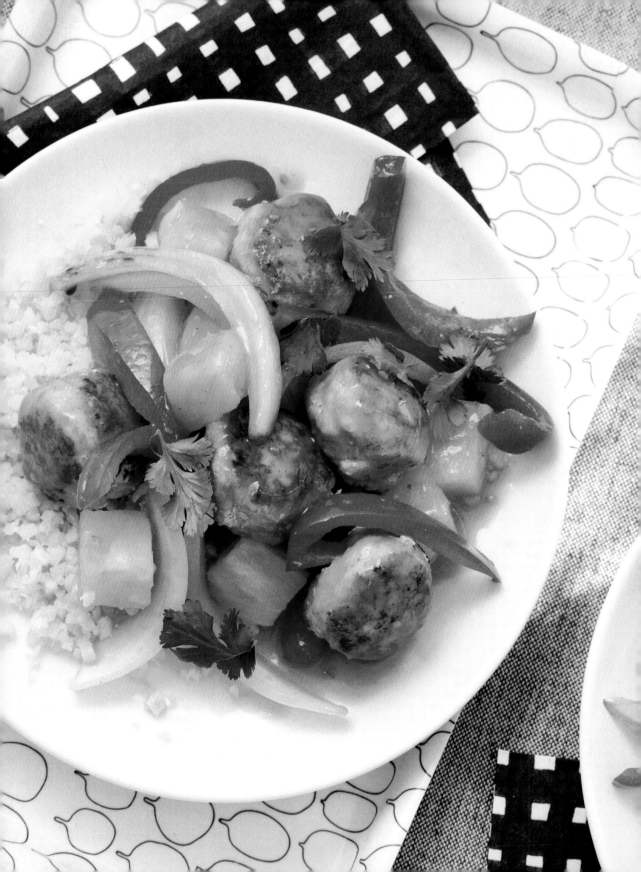

Sweet & Sour Chicken Meatballs

One 8-ounce can pineapple chunks packed in juice (not drained)

1½ teaspoons cornstarch

1½ tablespoons seasoned rice vinegar

1 tablespoon thick teriyaki sauce or marinade

8 ounces raw extra-lean ground chicken (at least 98% lean)

2 tablespoons (about 1 large) egg white or fat-free liquid egg substitute

2 tablespoons panko bread crumbs

¼ teaspoon garlic powder

¼ teaspoon ground ginger

⅛ teaspoon each salt and black pepper

1 cup sliced red bell pepper

1 cup sliced onion

Optional topping: fresh cilantro

Serving suggestion: riced cauliflower

 30m

Prep: 15 minutes

Cook: 15 minutes

You'll need:
medium bowl, large bowl, skillet with lid, nonstick spray

½ of recipe:
290 calories
2g total fat
(<0.5g sat fat)
762mg sodium
33.5g carbs
3g fiber
23g sugars
29g protein

290 calories

1. To make the sauce, drain the juice from the pineapple into a medium bowl. (Set pineapple chunks aside.) Add cornstarch, and stir to dissolve. Add vinegar and teriyaki, and mix until uniform.

2. In a large bowl, combine chicken, egg whites/substitute, panko, garlic powder, ginger, salt, and black pepper. Mix thoroughly, and firmly form into 10 meatballs.

3. Bring a skillet sprayed with nonstick spray to medium-high heat. Add meatballs, bell pepper, and onion. Cook until meatballs have browned on all sides and veggies have slightly softened, about 5 minutes, rotating meatballs and stirring veggies as you cook.

4. Reduce heat to medium low. Cover and cook for 5 minutes, or until meatballs are cooked through.

5. Add sauce and pineapple chunks. Cook and stir until sauce has thickened and entire dish is hot, about 1 minute.

MAKES 2 SERVINGS

Stir-Frys & Skillet Meals: Poultry

Quickie Chicken Piccata

I serve this one over riced cauliflower. It's also great over whole-wheat spaghetti. The perfect dinner!

1 tablespoon whipped butter
½ cup reduced-sodium chicken broth
1½ teaspoons cornstarch
¼ cup dry white wine
2 teaspoons lemon juice
Two 5-ounce raw boneless skinless chicken breast cutlets
¼ teaspoon each salt and black pepper
1 tablespoon capers, drained
Optional topping: fresh parsley

1. To make the sauce, place butter in a medium microwave-safe bowl. Microwave for 15 seconds, or until melted. Add broth and cornstarch, and stir to dissolve. Add wine and lemon juice, and mix well.

2. Bring a skillet sprayed with nonstick spray to medium heat. Add chicken, salt, and pepper. Cook for 4 minutes per side, or until fully cooked.

3. Add sauce and capers. Cook and stir until sauce has slightly thickened, about 3 minutes.

MAKES 2 SERVINGS

Prep: 10 minutes

Cook: 15 minutes

You'll need:
medium microwave-safe bowl, skillet, nonstick spray

½ of recipe:
237 calories
7g total fat
(2.5g sat fat)
619mg sodium
3.5g carbs
<0.5g fiber
0.5g sugars
32g protein

Stir-Frys & Skillet Meals: Poultry

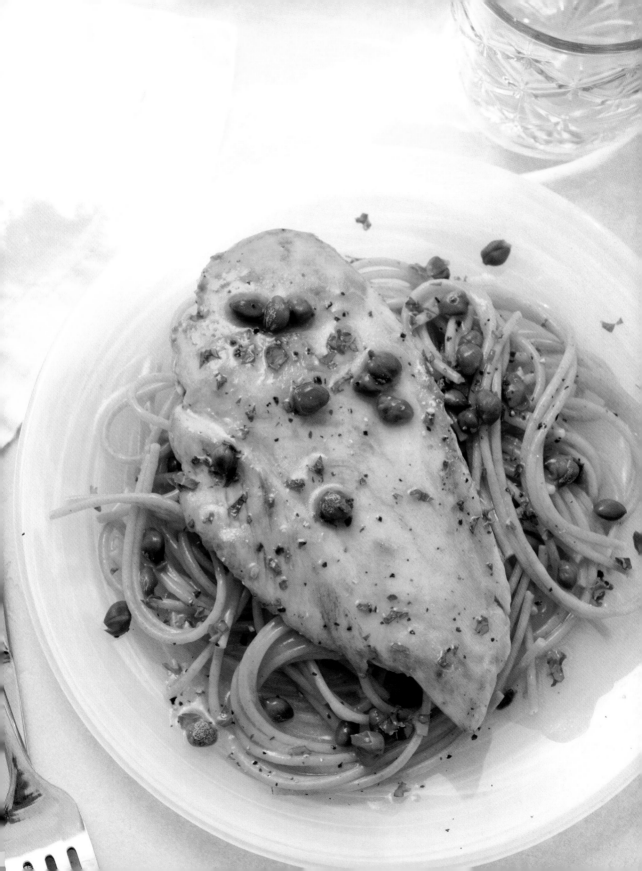

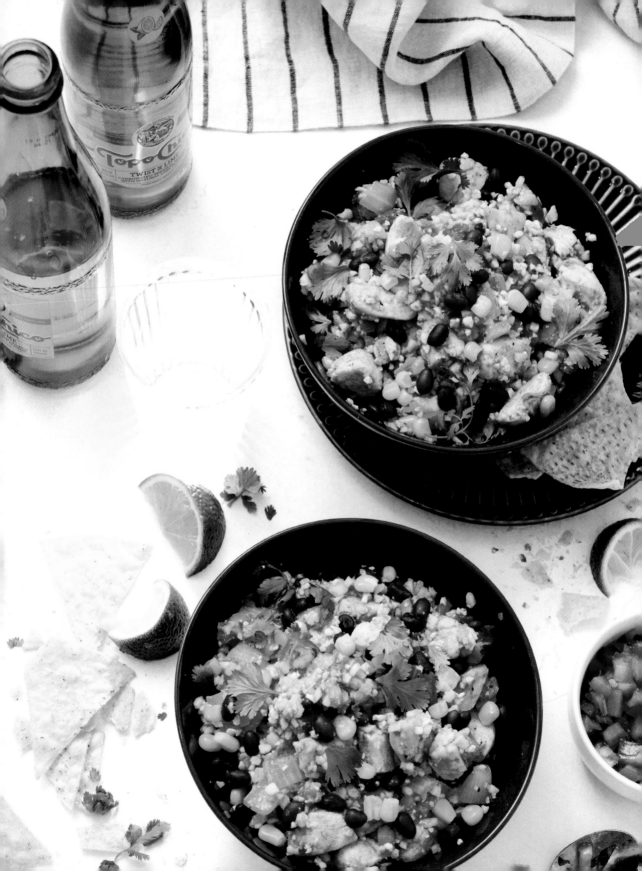

Southwestern Chicken Stir-Fry

8 ounces raw boneless skinless chicken breast, cut into bite-size pieces

1 cup chopped onion

⅛ teaspoon each salt and black pepper

3 cups frozen riced cauliflower

½ cup canned black beans, drained and rinsed

¼ cup frozen sweet corn kernels

1½ teaspoons taco seasoning

½ teaspoon garlic powder

¼ cup salsa

2 tablespoons chopped fresh cilantro

Prep: 10 minutes

Cook: 15 minutes

You'll need:
skillet with lid, nonstick spray

½ of recipe:
308 calories
4g total fat
(0.5g sat fat)
655mg sodium
34g carbs
9g fiber
10.5g sugars
34.5g protein

308 calories

1. Bring a skillet sprayed with nonstick spray to medium-high heat. Add chicken, onion, salt, and pepper. Cook and stir until onion has slightly softened, about 3 minutes.

2. Mix in cauliflower. Cover and cook for 5 minutes.

3. Add black beans, corn, taco seasoning, and garlic powder. Cook and stir until chicken is fully cooked and entire dish is hot, about 3 minutes.

4. Serve topped with salsa and cilantro.

MAKES 2 SERVINGS

Summer Chicken Sausage Stir-Fry

274 calories

The walnuts, the feta, the cranberries . . . This is one unexpected stir-fry, and it's insanely delicious.

Prep: 10 minutes

Cook: 10 minutes

You'll need:
skillet with lid, nonstick spray

½ of recipe:
274 calories
15g total fat
(4.5g total fat)
807mg sodium
17g carbs
3g fiber
11g sugars
19.5g protein

2 cups chopped kale
2 cups yellow squash sliced into coins
⅛ teaspoon salt and black pepper
6 ounces (about 2 links) fully cooked chicken sausage, sliced into coins
½ ounce (about 2 tablespoons) chopped walnuts
¼ cup crumbled feta cheese
2 tablespoons sweetened dried cranberries, chopped

1. Bring a skillet sprayed with nonstick spray to medium-high heat. Add kale and ¼ cup water. Cover and cook for 3 minutes, or until tender.

2. Add squash, salt, and pepper. Cook and stir until squash has slightly softened and any excess liquid has evaporated, about 3 minutes.

3. Add sausage and walnuts. Cook and stir until sausage has slightly browned and walnuts are hot, about 2 minutes.

4. Serve topped with feta and cranberries.

MAKES 2 SERVINGS

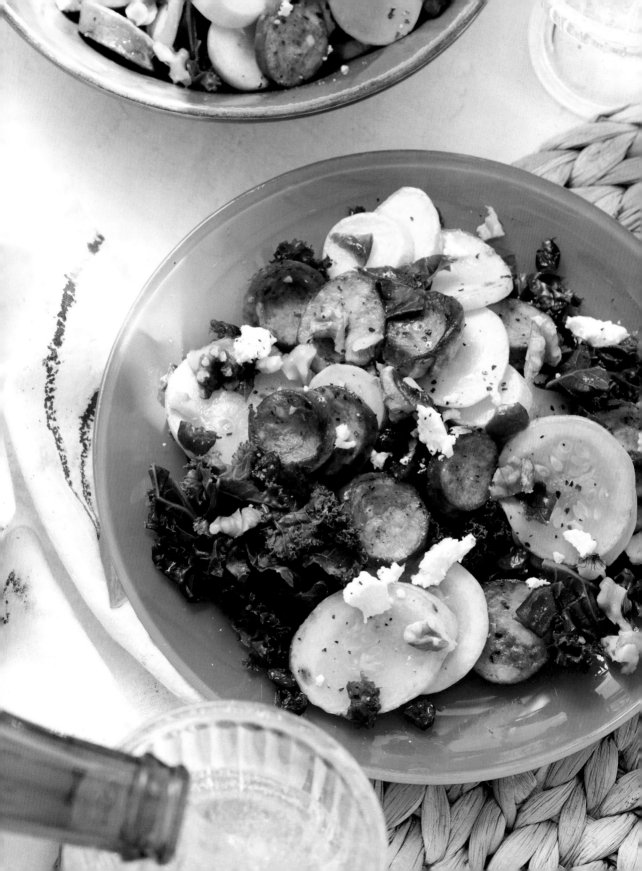

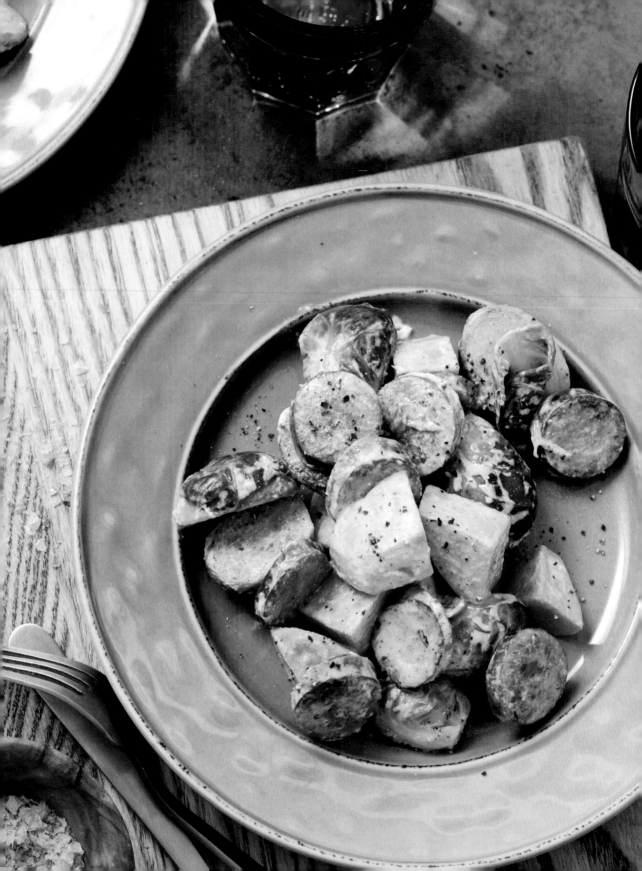

Autumn Chicken Sausage Stir-Fry

The combination of Dijon mustard and cream cheese is so delicious that it'll give you chills!

10 ounces (about 1 medium) sweet potato, peeled and cut into 1-inch cubes

8 ounces (about 16 medium) Brussels sprouts, trimmed and halved

6 ounces (about 2 links) fully cooked chicken sausage, sliced into coins

2 tablespoons light/reduced-fat cream cheese

1 tablespoon Dijon mustard

⅛ teaspoon garlic powder

⅛ teaspoon onion powder

1. Place sweet potato and Brussels sprouts in a large microwave-safe bowl with ¼ cup water. Cover and microwave for 6 minutes, or until mostly softened. Drain excess water.

2. Bring a skillet sprayed with nonstick spray to medium-high heat. Add sausage, sweet potato, and Brussels sprouts. Cook and stir until sausage has slightly browned and sweet potato and Brussels sprouts have softened, about 3 minutes.

3. Add cream cheese, mustard, garlic powder, and onion powder. Cook and stir until melted and well mixed, about 1 minute.

MAKES 2 SERVINGS

344 calories

Prep: 10 minutes

Cook: 15 minutes

You'll need:
large microwave-safe bowl, skillet, nonstick spray

½ of recipe:
344 calories
10g total fat
(4g sat fat)
811mg sodium
42.5g carbs
8.5g fiber
10.5g sugars
21g protein

Stir-Frys & Skillet Meals: Poultry

Thanksgiving Skillet

This recipe screams Thanksgiving! (Not literally. If your cookbook is shouting at you, then YOU should run screaming.)

Prep: 10 minutes

Cook: 15 minutes

You'll need:
skillet with lid, nonstick spray

½ of recipe:
308 calories
2.5g total fat
(0.5g sat fat)
591mg sodium
35.5g carbs
4g fiber
21.5g sugars
36.5g protein

Two 5-ounce raw boneless skinless turkey breast cutlets
⅛ teaspoon ground sage
⅛ teaspoon dried thyme
⅛ teaspoon each salt and black pepper
1½ cups chopped mushrooms
1 cup chopped Fuji or Gala apple
1 cup chopped onion
½ cup chicken or turkey gravy
¼ cup sweetened dried cranberries, chopped
Optional topping: fresh thyme

1. Bring a skillet sprayed with nonstick spray to medium heat. Add turkey and seasonings. Cook for 4 minutes per side, or until turkey is cooked through. Plate turkey, and cover to keep warm.

2. Remove skillet from heat, respray, and bring to medium-high heat. Add mushrooms, apple, and onion. Cover and cook for 4 minutes, or until mostly softened.

3. Remove lid. Cook and stir until liquid has evaporated, about 2 minutes.

4. Remove skillet from heat, and mix in gravy. Spoon mixture over the turkey, and top with cranberries.

MAKES 2 SERVINGS

HG Tip
If you like this recipe, chances are you'll love the Turkey & Cranberry Slaw on page 35!

Stir-Frys & Skillet Meals: Poultry

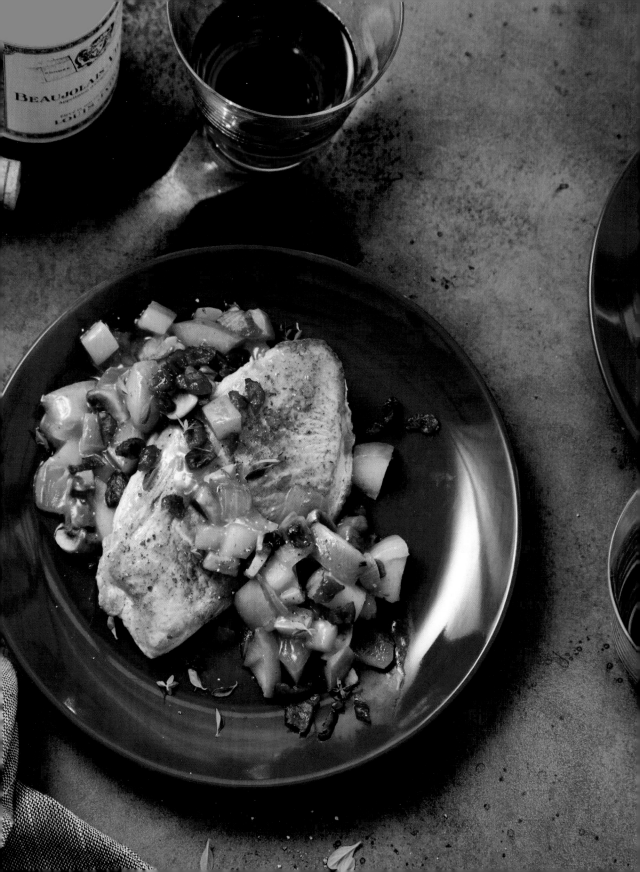

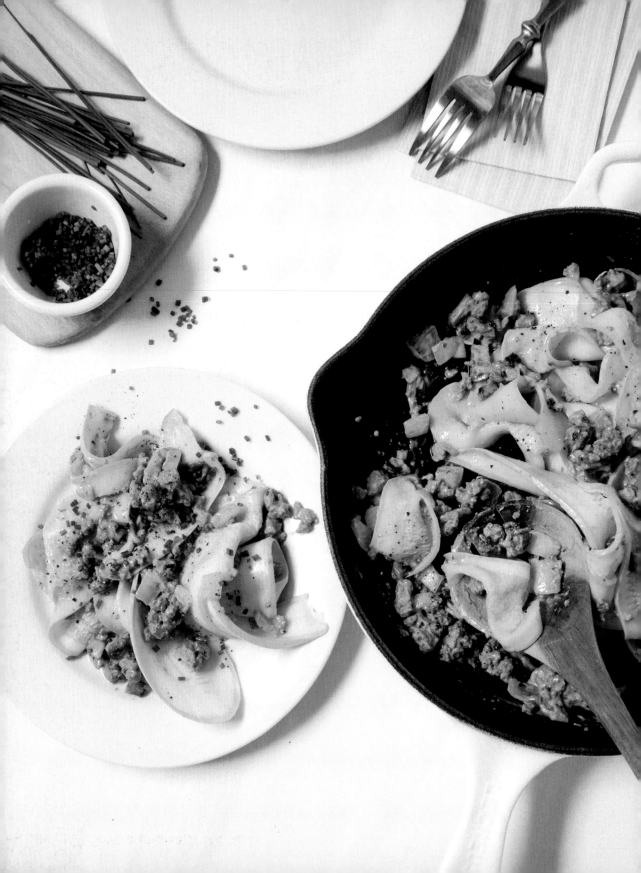

Ground Beef Stroganoff

These days, yellow squash peeled into wide noodles is one of my go-to pasta swaps. You don't even need a spiralizer!

2½ teaspoons au jus or brown gravy mix
1 tablespoon cornstarch
20 ounces (about 3 medium) yellow squash
8 ounces raw extra-lean ground beef (at least 96% lean)
1½ cups chopped mushrooms
1 cup chopped onion
¼ teaspoon garlic powder
¼ teaspoon onion powder
¼ cup light/reduced-fat cream cheese

1. In a small bowl, combine gravy mix, cornstarch, and 2 tablespoons water. Stir to dissolve.

2. Slice off and discard squash ends. Using a veggie peeler, slice squash into wide strips.

3. Bring a large skillet sprayed with nonstick spray to medium-high heat. Add squash, and cook and stir until slightly softened, about 4 minutes. Transfer to a strainer, and thoroughly drain.

4. Remove skillet from heat, respray, and return to medium-high heat. Add beef, mushrooms, onion, garlic powder, and onion powder. Cook and crumble until beef has browned and veggies have slightly softened, about 3 minutes.

5. Reduce heat to medium. Return squash to the skillet. Add gravy mixture and cream cheese. Cook and stir until beef is fully cooked, cream cheese has melted, and sauce has thickened, about 4 minutes.

MAKES 2 SERVINGS

Prep: 10 minutes

Cook: 15 minutes

You'll need:
small bowl,
veggie peeler,
large skillet,
nonstick spray,
strainer

½ of recipe:
331 calories
11.5g total fat
(6g sat fat)
663mg sodium
26.5g carbs
5g fiber
11.5g sugars
32g protein

331 calories

Stir-Frys & Skillet Meals: Beef & Pork

Breakfast for Dinner Omelette

317 calories

I love steak and I love egg-white omelettes, so why not combine the two?

4 ounces chopped raw lean flank steak
½ cup chopped onion
½ teaspoon garlic powder
½ teaspoon onion powder
⅛ teaspoon each salt and black pepper
Dash cumin
1 cup spinach
¾ cup (about 6 large) egg whites or fat-free liquid egg substitute
Optional topping: everything bagel seasoning

1. Bring a skillet sprayed with nonstick spray to medium-high heat. Add steak, onion, ¼ teaspoon garlic powder, ¼ teaspoon onion powder, salt, pepper, and cumin. Cook and stir until steak is fully cooked and onion has slightly softened, about 3 minutes.

2. Add spinach, and cook and stir until wilted, about 1 minute. Transfer to a medium bowl, and cover to keep warm.

3. Remove skillet from heat, respray, and bring to medium heat. Add egg whites/substitute and remaining ¼ teaspoon each garlic powder and onion powder. Cover and cook for 4 minutes, or until just set.

4. Top half of the omelette with the steak mixture, and fold the other half over the filling.

MAKES 1 SERVING

Prep: 10 minutes

Cook: 10 minutes

You'll need:
skillet with lid, nonstick spray, medium bowl

Entire recipe:
317 calories
7.5g total fat
(3g sat fat)
707mg sodium
12.5g carbs
2g fiber
4.5g sugars
47g protein

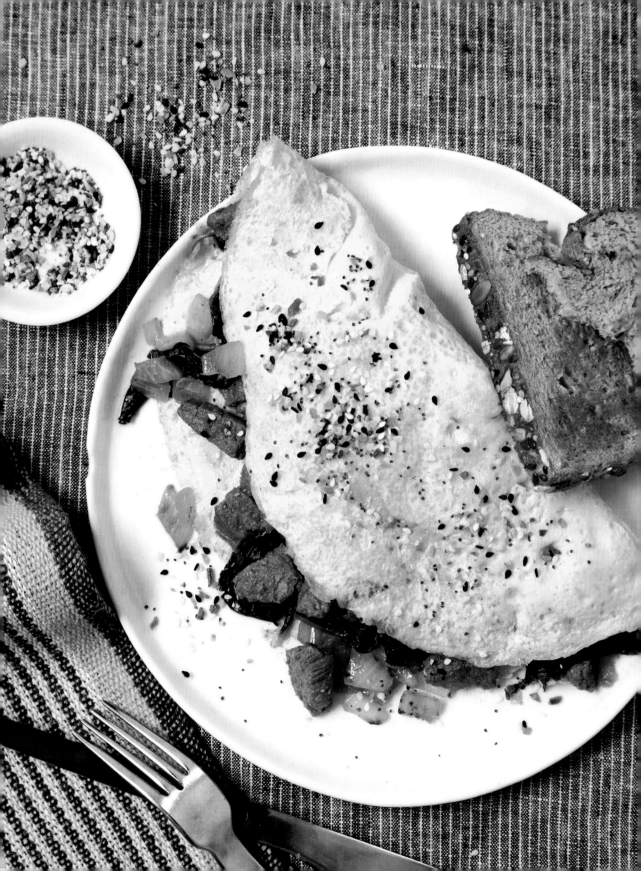

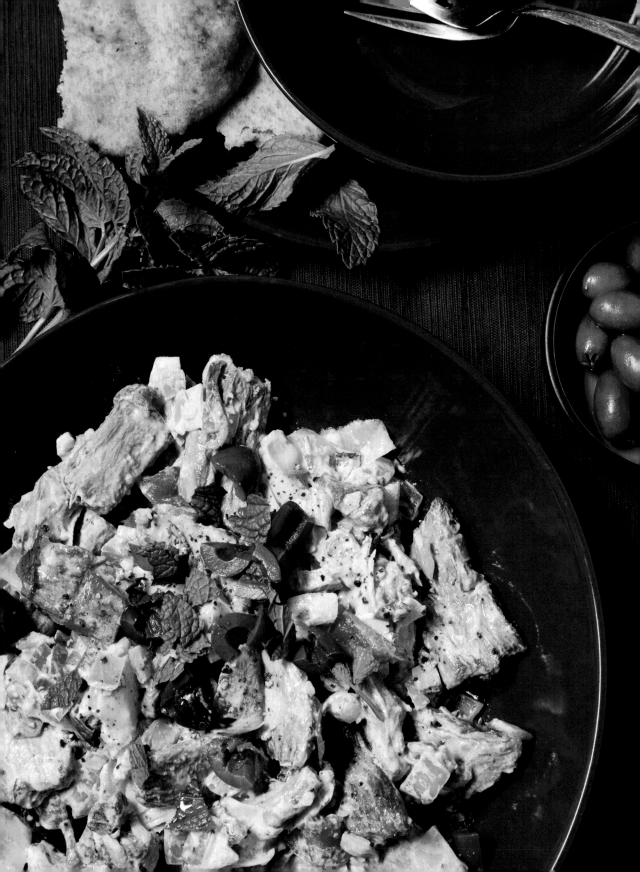

Mediterranean Steak Stir-Fry

¼ cup fat-free plain Greek yogurt

1 teaspoon chopped garlic

1 teaspoon chopped fresh mint

8 ounces thinly sliced raw lean flank steak

½ cup chopped red onion

¼ teaspoon garlic powder

¼ teaspoon onion powder

¼ teaspoon dried oregano

⅛ teaspoon each salt and black pepper

½ cup canned artichoke hearts packed in water, drained and chopped

¼ cup roasted red peppers packed in water, drained and chopped

2 tablespoons sliced black or Kalamata olives

1. In a medium bowl, combine yogurt, garlic, and mint. Mix well.

2. Bring a skillet sprayed with nonstick spray to medium-high heat. Add steak, onion, and seasonings. Cook and stir until steak is fully cooked and onion has slightly softened, about 3 minutes.

3. Reduce heat to medium low. Add artichokes, red peppers, and yogurt mixture. Cook and stir until hot and well mixed, about 2 minutes.

4. Serve topped with olives.

MAKES 2 SERVINGS

15m GF

247 calories

Prep: 10 minutes

Cook: 5 minutes

You'll need:
medium bowl, skillet, nonstick spray

½ of recipe:
247 calories
8.5g total fat
(3g sat fat)
576mg sodium
11.5g carbs
2.5g fiber
4.5g sugars
29g protein

Stir-Frys & Skillet Meals: Beef & Pork

Steak Teriyaki Stir-Fry

Any garlic fans in the house? This stir-fry will make you VERY happy . . .

2 cups frozen broccoli florets
1 cup sliced red bell pepper
1 cup sugar snap peas
8 ounces thinly sliced raw lean flank steak
2 tablespoons thick teriyaki sauce or marinade
1 tablespoon reduced-sodium/lite soy sauce
1 tablespoon chopped garlic

1. Bring a large skillet sprayed with nonstick spray to medium-high heat. Add broccoli, pepper, sugar snap peas, and 2 tablespoons water. Cover and cook for 5 minutes, or until broccoli has thawed and veggies are hot.

2. Add steak, and cook and stir until veggies have softened and steak is cooked through, about 4 minutes.

3. Stir in teriyaki, soy sauce, and garlic.

MAKES 2 SERVINGS

30m

Prep: 10 minutes

Cook: 10 minutes

You'll need:
large skillet with lid, nonstick spray

½ of recipe:
263 calories
7.5g total fat
(3g sat fat)
767mg sodium
17g carbs
4g fiber
9g sugars
29g protein

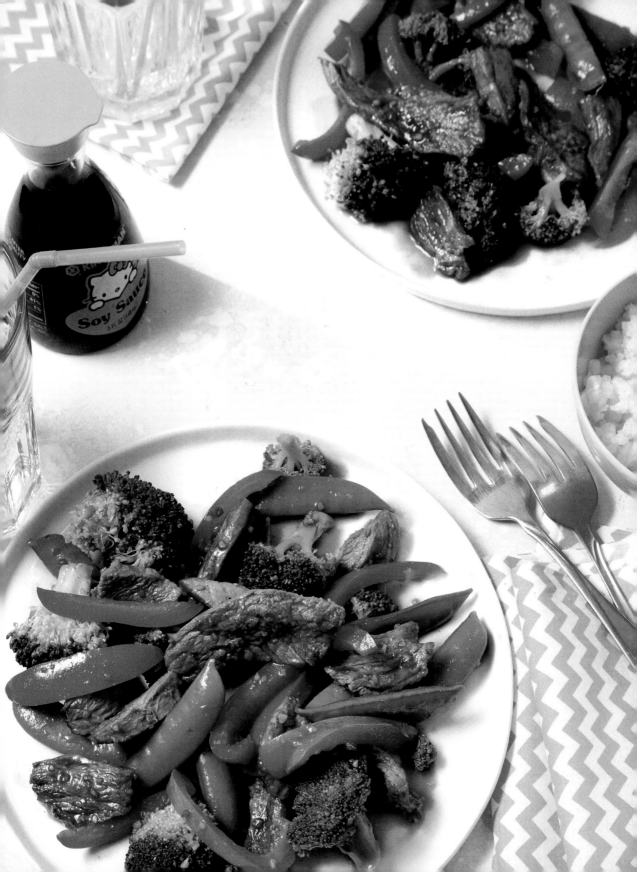

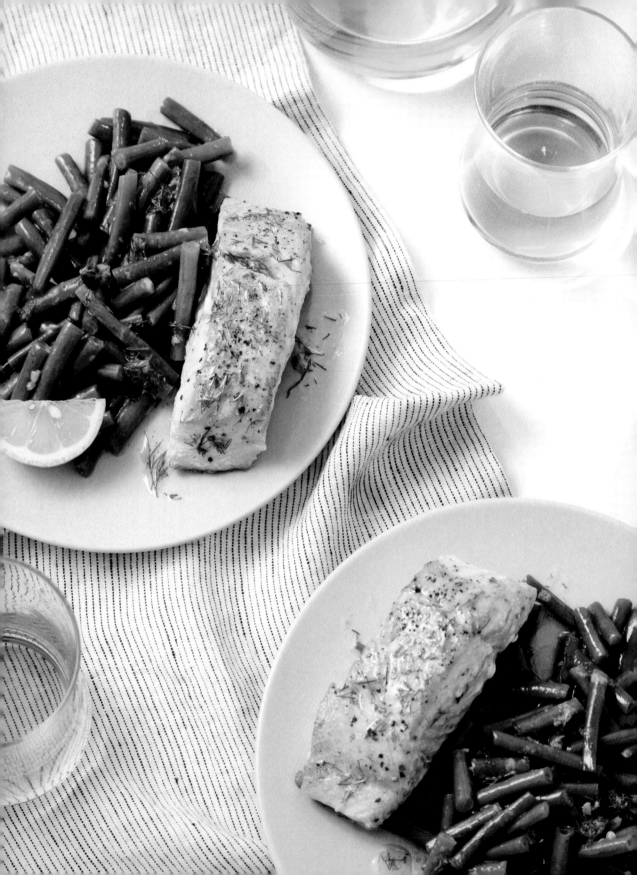

Pan-Seared Lemon & Dill Salmon

Salmon is one of my favorites, and this is such a simple way to prepare it. So fast, easy, and fresh!

2 cups green beans cut into 1-inch pieces
Two 4-ounce raw skinless salmon fillets
¼ teaspoon each salt and black pepper
2 tablespoons whipped butter
1 tablespoon lemon juice
1 tablespoon finely chopped fresh dill
2 teaspoons chopped garlic

1. Bring a large skillet sprayed with nonstick spray to medium-high heat. Add green beans and 2 tablespoons water. Cover and cook for 4 minutes, or until partly softened.

2. Add salmon, salt, and pepper. Stirring occasionally, cook until green beans have softened and salmon is cooked through, about 4 minutes per side. Plate salmon and green beans.

3. Reduce heat to low. Add butter, lemon juice, dill, and garlic. Cook and stir until melted and well mixed, about 1 minute. Spoon sauce over salmon and green beans.

MAKES 2 SERVINGS

282 calories

Prep: 5 minutes

Cook: 15 minutes

You'll need:
large skillet with lid, nonstick spray

½ of recipe:
282 calories
16g total fat
(6g sat fat)
426mg sodium
9.5g carbs
4g fiber
1.5g sugars
25.5g protein

Stir-Frys & Skillet Meals: Seafood

Honey-Lime Shrimp

293
calories

2 cups sliced bell peppers

2 cups frozen broccoli florets

8 ounces (about 16) raw large shrimp, peeled, tails removed, deveined

2 tablespoons whipped butter

2 tablespoons honey

1 tablespoon chopped garlic

1 tablespoon lime juice

⅛ teaspoon each salt and black pepper

1. Bring a large skillet sprayed with nonstick spray to medium-high heat. Add bell peppers, broccoli, and 2 tablespoons water. Cover and cook for 5 minutes, or until broccoli has thawed and veggies are hot.

2. Add shrimp. Cook and stir until veggies have softened and shrimp are fully cooked, about 4 minutes.

3. Reduce heat to low. Add butter, honey, garlic, lime juice, salt, and black pepper. Cook and stir until melted and well mixed, about 1 minute.

MAKES 2 SERVINGS

Prep: 10 minutes

Cook: 10 minutes

You'll need:
large skillet with lid, nonstick spray

**½ of recipe
(about 1¾ cups):**
293 calories
8g total fat
(4g sat fat)
558mg sodium
29.5g carbs
4g fiber
22.5g sugars
24g protein

Stir-Frys & Skillet Meals: Seafood

Hungry Girl *FAST* & *Easy*

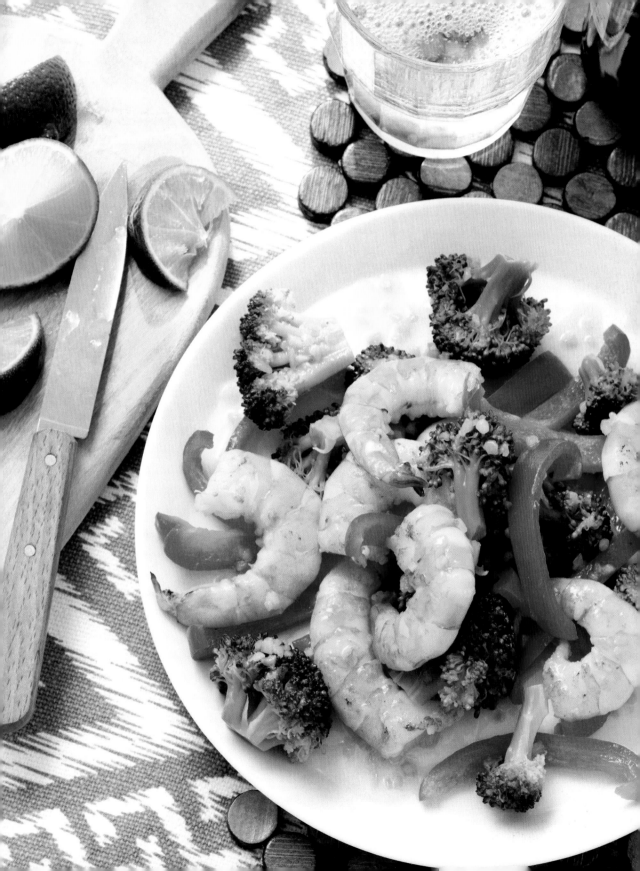

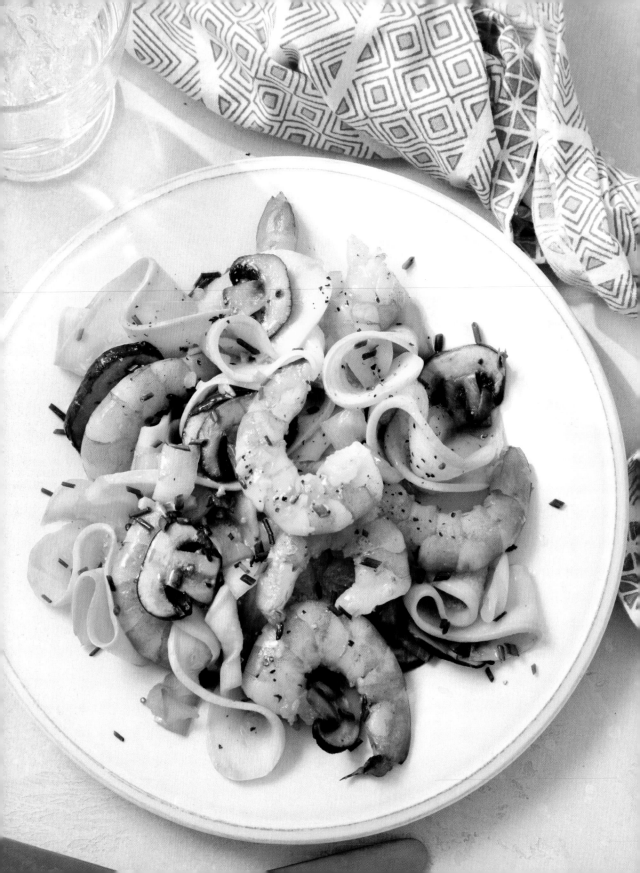

Garlic-Butter Shrimp with Squash Noodles

This pasta swap is so good, you could fool someone into thinking it's made with real noodles.

20 ounces (about 2 medium) yellow squash
2 cups sliced brown mushrooms
1 cup chopped onion
8 ounces (about 16) raw large shrimp, peeled, tails removed, deveined
2 tablespoons whipped butter
1 tablespoon chopped garlic
1 tablespoon lemon juice
Dash each salt and black pepper
Optional topping: fresh chives

1. Slice off and discard squash ends. Using a veggie peeler, slice squash into wide strips.

2. Bring a large skillet sprayed with nonstick spray to medium-high heat. Add squash, and cook and stir until slightly softened, about 4 minutes. Transfer to a strainer, and thoroughly drain.

3. Remove skillet from heat, respray, and return to medium-high heat. Add mushrooms and onion. Cook and stir until slightly softened and lightly browned, about 3 minutes.

4. Add shrimp, butter, garlic, lemon juice, salt, and pepper. Cook and stir until veggies have softened and shrimp are cooked through, about 3 minutes.

5. Return squash to the skillet, and cook and stir until hot and well mixed, about 2 minutes.

MAKES 2 SERVINGS

Prep: 15 minutes

Cook: 15 minutes

270 calories

You'll need:
veggie peeler,
large skillet,
nonstick spray,
strainer

½ of recipe:
270 calories
8.5g total fat
(4g sat fat)
479mg sodium
22g carbs
5g fiber
12g sugars
27g protein

Stir-Frys & Skillet Meals: Seafood

Creamy Cajun Shrimp

235 calories

Fire-roasted tomatoes + cream cheese + Cajun seasoning = a total game changer!

2 cups sliced bell peppers
1 cup sliced onion
8 ounces (about 16) raw large shrimp, peeled, tails removed, deveined
2 teaspoons lime juice
½ teaspoon garlic powder
½ cup canned fire-roasted diced tomatoes, lightly drained
¼ cup light/reduced-fat cream cheese
1 teaspoon Cajun seasoning

1. Bring a skillet sprayed with nonstick spray to medium-high heat. Add peppers and onion. Cook and stir until slightly softened and lightly browned, about 4 minutes.

2. Add shrimp, lime juice, and garlic powder. Cook and stir until veggies have softened and shrimp are fully cooked, about 4 minutes.

3. Reduce heat to medium-low. Add tomatoes, cream cheese, and Cajun seasoning. Cook and stir until melted and well mixed, about 1 minute.

MAKES 2 SERVINGS

Prep: 10 minutes

Cook: 10 minutes

You'll need:
skillet, nonstick spray

½ of recipe:
235 calories
7g total fat
(4g sat fat)
730mg sodium
17g carbs
3.5g fiber
8.5g sugars
25g protein

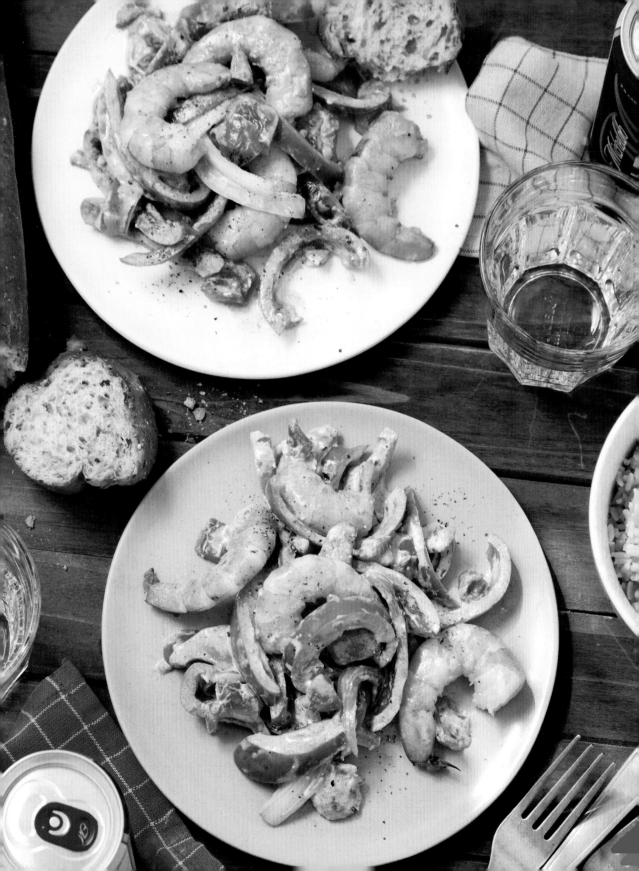

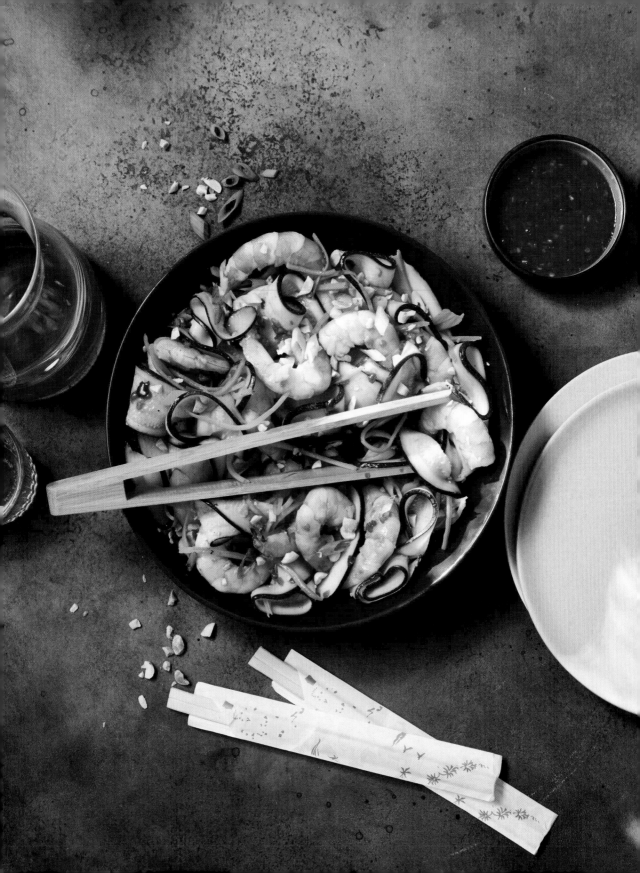

1 tablespoon reduced-sodium/lite soy sauce

1 tablespoon sweet chili sauce

1½ teaspoons lime juice

1 teaspoon sesame oil

1 teaspoon chopped garlic

20 ounces (about 2 large) zucchini

1 cup shredded carrots

8 ounces (about 16) raw large shrimp, peeled, tails removed, deveined

⅓ cup chopped scallions

½ ounce (about 2 tablespoons) chopped peanuts

Optional topping: chopped fresh cilantro

1. In a small bowl, combine soy sauce, chili sauce, lime juice, oil, and garlic. Mix until uniform.

2. Slice off and discard zucchini ends. Using a veggie peeler, slice zucchini into wide strips.

3. Bring a large skillet sprayed with nonstick spray to medium-high heat. Add zucchini and carrots. Cook and stir until hot and slightly softened, about 3 minutes. Transfer to a strainer, and thoroughly drain.

4. Remove skillet from heat, respray, and return to medium-high heat. Add shrimp, and cook and stir until cooked through, about 4 minutes.

5. Reduce heat to medium-low. Add drained veggies and sauce mixture. Cook and stir until hot and well mixed, about 2 minutes.

6. Serve topped with scallions and peanuts.

MAKES 2 SERVINGS

30m

Prep: 15 minutes

Cook: 10 minutes

You'll need:
small bowl,
veggie peeler,
large skillet,
nonstick spray,
strainer

½ of recipe:
270 calories
8g total fat
(1g sat fat)
795mg sodium
23.5g carbs
5.5g fiber
15g sugars
27.5g protein

270 calories

Stir-Frys & Skillet Meals: Seafood

Scallop Scampi

243 calories

Broccoli slaw does it again. You get so many tasty veggies with minimal effort!

Prep: 5 minutes

Cook: 15 minutes

You'll need:
large microwave-safe bowl, skillet with lid, nonstick spray

½ of recipe:
243 calories
10g total fat
(5.5g sat fat)
778mg sodium
16g carbs
4g fiber
4.5g sugars
19.5g protein

4 cups bagged broccoli slaw
8 ounces (about 6) raw large scallops
⅛ teaspoon each salt and black pepper
2½ tablespoons whipped butter
2 tablespoons dry white wine
1 tablespoon chopped garlic
1 tablespoon lemon juice
1 tablespoon grated Parmesan cheese

1. Place broccoli slaw in a large microwave-safe bowl with ¼ cup water. Cover and microwave for 5 minutes, or until softened. Drain excess liquid, and cover to keep warm.

2. Bring a skillet sprayed with nonstick spray to medium-high heat. Add scallops, salt, and pepper. Cook for 2 minutes per side, until fully cooked.

3. Reduce heat to medium-low. Add butter, wine, garlic, and lemon juice. Cook and stir until melted and well mixed, about 1 minute.

4. Spoon sauce and scallops over the broccoli slaw, and sprinkle with Parm.

MAKES 2 SERVINGS

HG Tip
Keep an eye on your scallops so they don't overcook. Scallops are perfectly done when lightly browned and opaque.

Stir-Frys & Skillet Meals: Seafood

Hungry Girl *FAST* & Easy

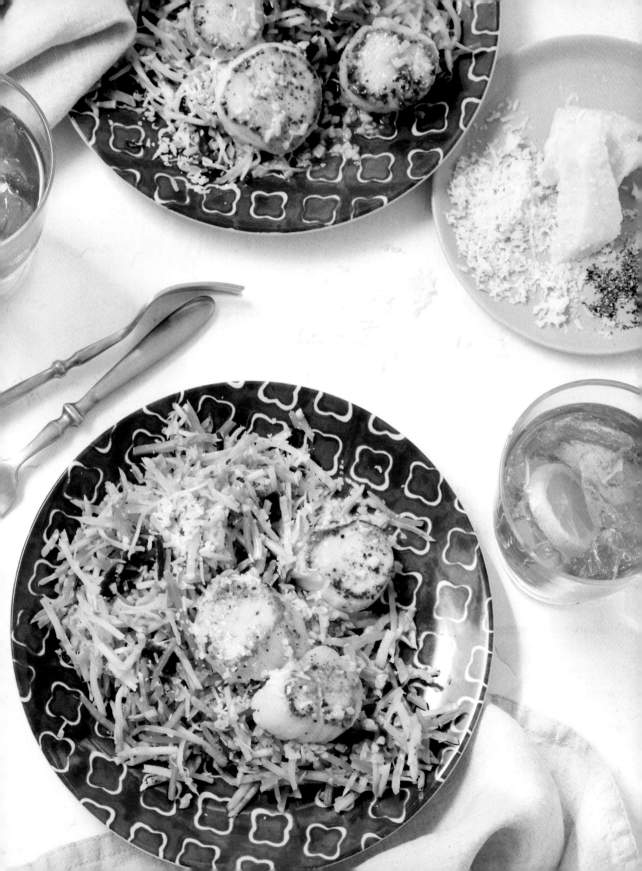

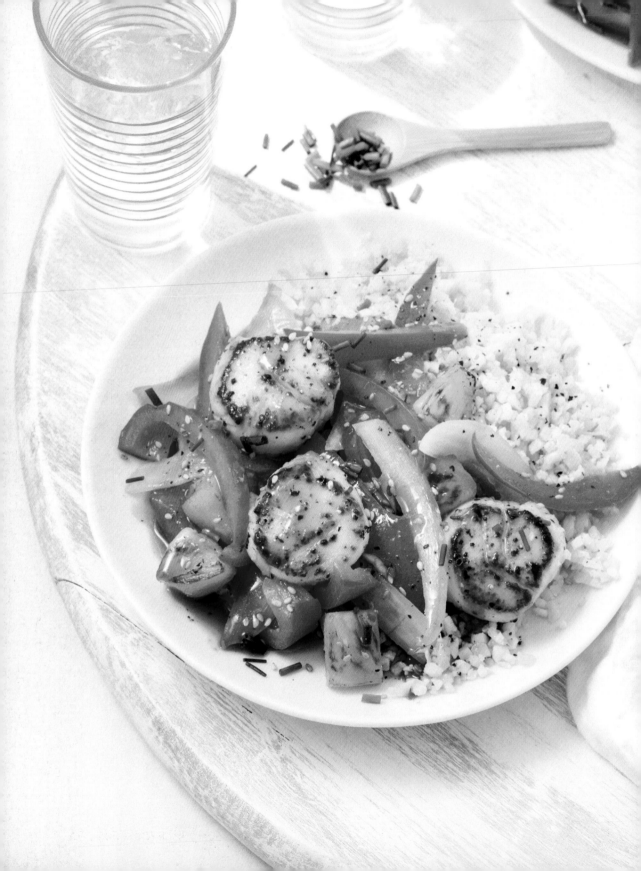

This dish was inspired by the pineapple chicken my mom used to make. Turns out, pineapple & teriyaki are just as good with scallops as they are with poultry!

½ cup pineapple chunks packed in juice (not drained)
2 tablespoons thick teriyaki sauce or marinade
2 cups sliced red bell peppers
2 cups sliced onion
8 ounces (about 6) raw large scallops
Optional topping: fresh chives
Serving suggestion: riced cauliflower

1. To make the sauce, drain juice (about 2 tablespoons) from the pineapple into a small bowl. (Set pineapple chunks aside.) Add teriyaki, and stir until uniform.

2. Bring a large skillet sprayed with nonstick spray to medium-high heat. Add peppers and onion. Cook and stir until slightly softened, about 3 minutes.

3. Add scallops. Cook and stir until veggies have softened and scallops are cooked through, about 4 minutes.

4. Add sauce and pineapple chunks, and cook and stir until hot and well mixed, about 1 minute.

MAKES 2 SERVINGS

Prep: 5 minutes

Cook: 10 minutes

You'll need:
small bowl, large skillet, nonstick spray

½ of recipe:
208 calories
1g total fat
(<0.5g sat fat)
863mg sodium
32.5g carbs
5g fiber
19.5g sugars
16g protein

208 calories

Stir-Frys & Skillet Meals: Seafood

Scallops Faux-sotto

268 calories

20-minute risotto without the excess starchy carbs? You're welcome!

1 cup sliced brown mushrooms
1 cup chopped onion
1 tablespoon chopped garlic
1 teaspoon onion powder
3 cups frozen riced cauliflower
¼ cup light/reduced-fat cream cheese
1 tablespoon grated Parmesan cheese
8 ounces (about 6) raw large scallops
1 teaspoon lemon juice
Dash each salt and black pepper
Optional topping: fresh thyme

1. Bring a large skillet sprayed with nonstick spray to medium-high heat. Add mushrooms, onion, garlic, and onion powder. Cook and stir until slightly softened, about 2 minutes.

2. Add cauliflower, and cook and stir until fresh veggies have softened and cauliflower is hot, about 3 minutes.

3. Reduce heat to medium-low. Add cream cheese and Parm. Cook and stir until melted and well mixed, about 2 minutes. Transfer to a large bowl, and cover to keep warm.

4. Remove skillet from heat. Clean, if needed. Respray, and return to medium-high heat. Add scallops, lemon juice, salt, and pepper. Cook for 2 minutes per side, or until fully cooked.

5. Serve scallops over the cauliflower mixture.

MAKES 2 SERVINGS

Prep: 5 minutes

Cook: 15 minutes

You'll need:
large skillet,
nonstick spray,
large bowl

½ of recipe:
268 calories
8.5g total fat
(4.5g sat fat)
789mg sodium
27g carbs
6g fiber
10g sugars
24g protein

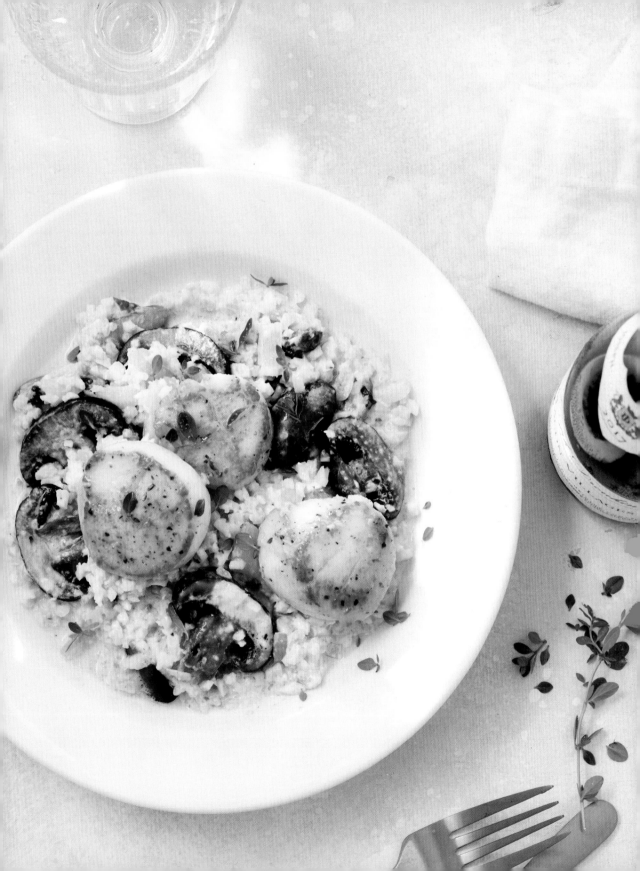

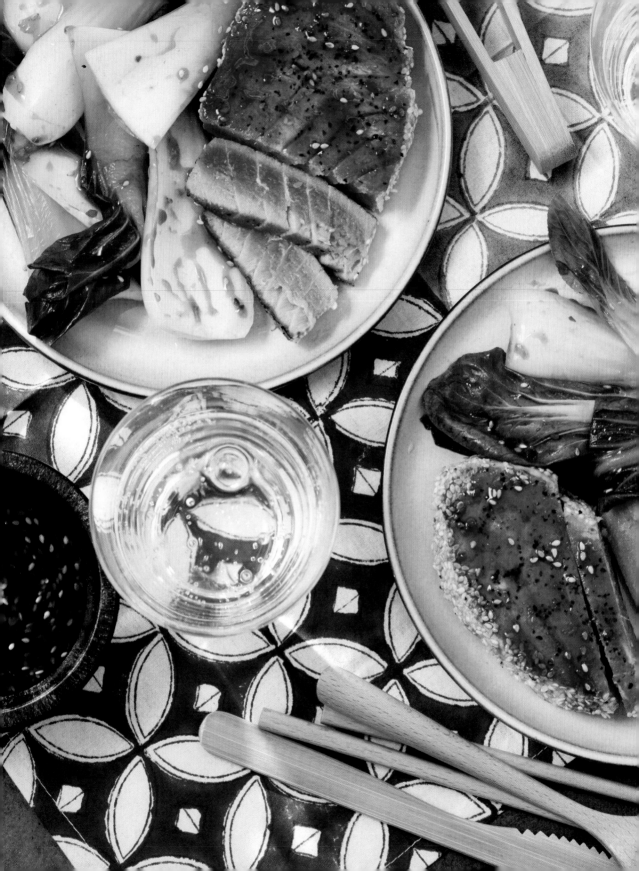

8 ounces (about 8 pieces) baby bok choy, ends trimmed
Two 5-ounce raw ahi/yellowfin tuna fillets
⅛ teaspoon each salt and black pepper
1 tablespoon sesame seeds
2 teaspoons sesame oil
1 tablespoon sweet chili sauce
1 tablespoon thick teriyaki sauce or marinade
Optional topping: chopped scallions

15m

266 calories

Prep: 5 minutes

Cook: 10 minutes

You'll need:
skillet with lid,
nonstick spray,
small bowl

½ of recipe:
266 calories
8g total fat
(1g sat fat)
609mg sodium
11g carbs
1.5g fiber
7g sugars
36g protein

1. Bring a skillet sprayed with nonstick spray to medium-high heat. Add bok choy and ¼ cup water. Cover and cook for 5 minutes, or until tender. Plate boy choy, and cover to keep warm.

2. Season tuna with salt and pepper. Coat edges with sesame seeds, lightly pressing to adhere.

3. Respray skillet, drizzle with oil, and return to medium-high heat. Add tuna, and cook for 2 minutes per side, or until cooked to your preference.

4. In a small bowl, mix chili sauce with teriyaki. Drizzle over tuna and bok choy.

MAKES 2 SERVINGS

Veggie Cashew Stir-Fry

225
calories

½ cup vegetable broth

2 teaspoons cornstarch

1 tablespoon seasoned rice vinegar

1½ teaspoons sweet chili sauce

1½ teaspoons reduced-sodium/lite soy sauce

½ teaspoon garlic powder

¼ teaspoon ground ginger

3 cups frozen broccoli florets

2 cups frozen stir-fry vegetables

2 cups quartered mushrooms

1 ounce (about ¼ cup) cashews

1. To make the sauce, in a medium bowl, combine broth with cornstarch. Stir to dissolve. Add vinegar, chili sauce, soy sauce, garlic powder, and ginger. Mix well.

2. Bring a large skillet sprayed with nonstick spray to medium-high heat. Add broccoli, stir-fry vegetables, and mushrooms. Cover and cook for 5 minutes, or until thawed.

3. Reduce heat to medium-low. Add cashews and sauce. Cook and stir until sauce has slightly thickened and coated the veggies, about 3 minutes.

MAKES 2 SERVINGS

Prep: 5 minutes

Cook: 10 minutes

You'll need:
medium bowl, large skillet with lid, nonstick spray

½ of recipe:
225 calories
6.5g total fat
(1g sat fat)
622mg sodium
29.5g carbs
6.5g fiber
13.5g sugars
9.5g protein

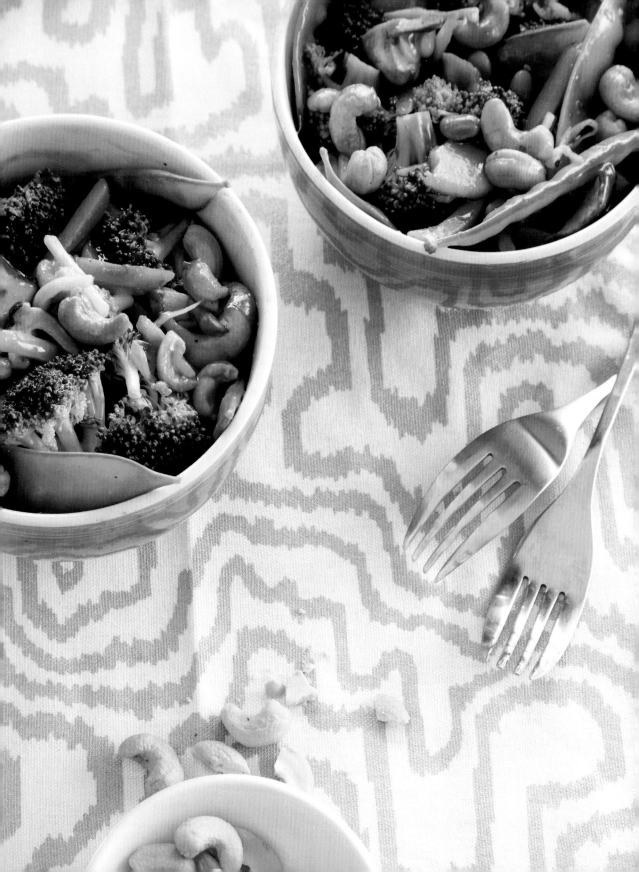

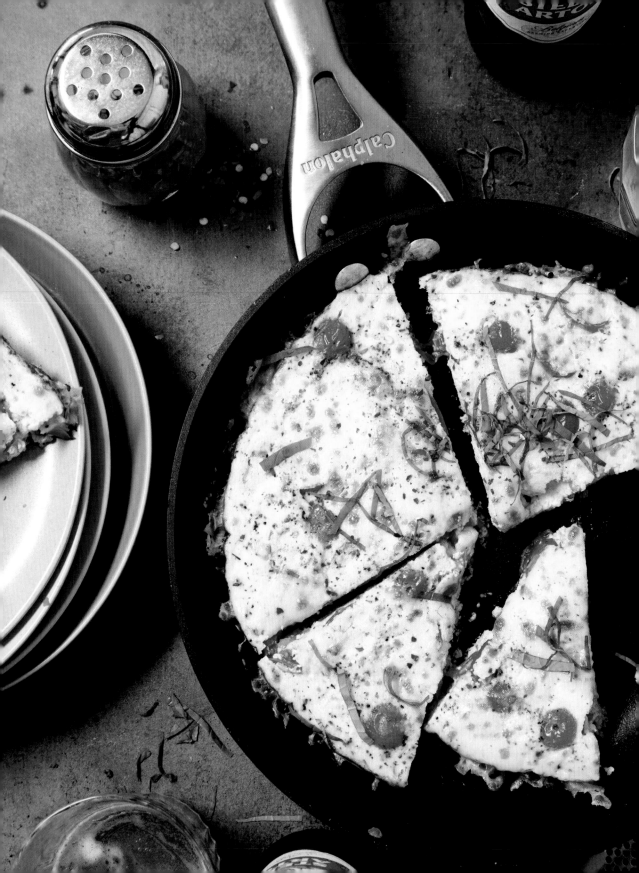

White Pizza Frittata

Whipping up a frittata is really SO easy. Once you get the process down, you'll want to frittata everything!

2 cups (about 16 large) egg whites or fat-free liquid egg substitute
¾ cup light/low-fat ricotta cheese
1 teaspoon garlic powder
¼ teaspoon Italian seasoning
¼ teaspoon each salt and black pepper
1½ cups cherry tomatoes, halved
½ cup shredded part-skim mozzarella cheese
Optional topping: chopped fresh basil, crushed red pepper flakes

1. Preheat broiler.

2. In a large bowl, combine egg whites/substitute, ricotta, and seasonings. Mix until smooth and uniform.

3. Bring a large oven-safe skillet sprayed with nonstick spray to medium heat. Add tomatoes, and cook and stir until softened, about 3 minutes.

4. Add egg mixture to the skillet, and gently stir so it coats the bottom. Cover and cook for 7 minutes, or until set.

5. Sprinkle with mozzarella. Broil until melted, about 3 minutes.

MAKES 4 SERVINGS

161 calories

Prep: 5 minutes

Cook: 15 minutes

You'll need:
large bowl, large oven-safe skillet with lid, nonstick spray

¼th of frittata:
161 calories
4.5g total fat
(3g sat fat)
518mg sodium
7g carbs
1g fiber
4g sugars
21.5g protein

Stir-Frys & Skillet Meals: Meatless

Very Veggie & Cheddar Frittata

188 calories

2 cups (about 16 large) egg whites or fat-free liquid egg substitute

1 cup shredded reduced-fat cheddar cheese

1 teaspoon garlic powder

¼ teaspoon plus ⅛ teaspoon each salt and black pepper

1 cup chopped bell peppers

1 cup chopped mushrooms

1 cup chopped onion

1 cup chopped zucchini

1. Preheat broiler.

2. In a large bowl, combine egg whites/substitute, ½ cup cheese, garlic powder, and ¼ teaspoon each salt and black pepper. Mix until uniform.

3. Bring a large oven-safe skillet sprayed with nonstick spray to medium-high heat. Add veggies and remaining ⅛ teaspoon each salt and black pepper. Cook and stir until softened, about 6 minutes.

4. Reduce heat to medium. Add egg mixture to the skillet, and gently stir so it coats the bottom. Cover and cook for 7 minutes, or until set.

5. Top with remaining ½ cup cheese. Broil until melted, about 3 minutes.

MAKES 4 SERVINGS

Prep: 10 minutes

Cook: 20 minutes

You'll need:
large bowl, large oven-safe skillet with lid, nonstick spray

¼th of frittata:
188 calories
6g total fat
(3.5g sat fat)
646mg sodium
10.5g carbs
2g fiber
4.5g sugars
22g protein

Stir-Frys & Skillet Meals: Meatless

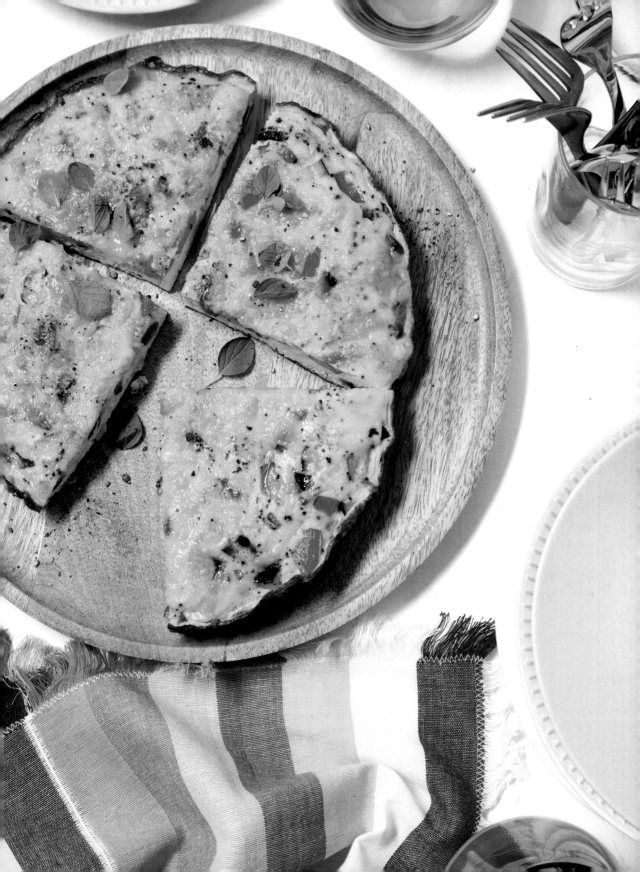

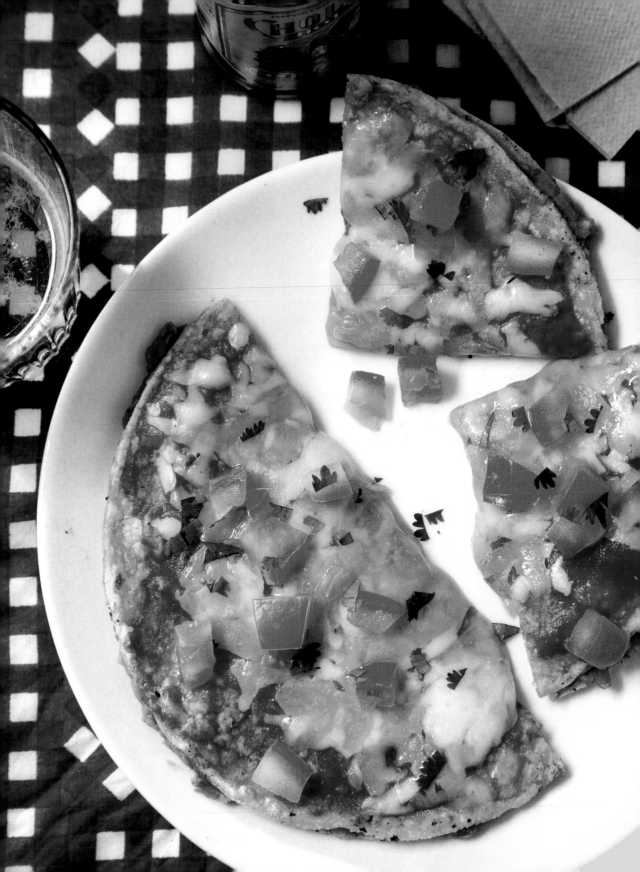

Skillet Mexican Pizza

Two 6-inch corn tortillas
⅓ cup fat-free refried beans
¼ teaspoon taco seasoning
1½ tablespoons taco sauce
3 tablespoons shredded reduced-fat Mexican-blend cheese
¼ cup chopped tomato

1. Bring a skillet sprayed with nonstick spray to medium-high heat. Add 1 tortilla, and cook until lightly browned, about 2 minutes.

2. Flip tortilla, and carefully spread with refried beans. Sprinkle with taco seasoning. Top with the other tortilla, followed by sauce, cheese, and tomato.

3. Cover and cook for 1 minute, or until cheese has melted and entire dish is hot.

MAKES 1 SERVING

5i **15m** **V** **GF**

253 calories

Prep: 5 minutes

Cook: 5 minutes

You'll need:
skillet with lid, nonstick spray

Entire recipe:
253 calories
5.5g total fat
(2.5g sat fat)
759mg sodium
38.5g carbs
7g fiber
3g sugars
12.5g protein

Stir-Frys & Skillet Meals: Meatless

Spicy Eggplant Stir-Fry

275 calories

Frozen edamame is such a smart ingredient for speedy meatless meals. It comes fully cooked, and just half a cup has 10g protein!

Prep: 5 minutes

Cook: 15 minutes

You'll need:
large skillet, nonstick spray, medium bowl

½ of recipe:
275 calories
8g total fat
(1g sat fat)
688mg sodium
38g carbs
13g fiber
20.5g sugars
14g protein

6 cups (about 1 large) cubed eggplant
⅛ teaspoon each salt and black pepper
2 cups snow peas
1 cup frozen shelled edamame
2 tablespoons sweet chili sauce
1 tablespoon reduced-sodium/lite soy sauce
2 teaspoons sesame oil
¼ teaspoon crushed red pepper
¼ teaspoon garlic powder

1. Bring a large skillet sprayed with nonstick spray to medium-high heat. Add eggplant, salt, and black pepper. Cook and stir until mostly softened, about 5 minutes.

2. Add snow peas and edamame. Cook and stir until fresh veggies have softened and edamame is hot, about 4 minutes.

3. Reduce heat to medium low. Add remaining ingredients. Cook and stir until hot and well mixed, about 1 minute.

MAKES 2 SERVINGS

Stir-Frys & Skillet Meals: Meatless

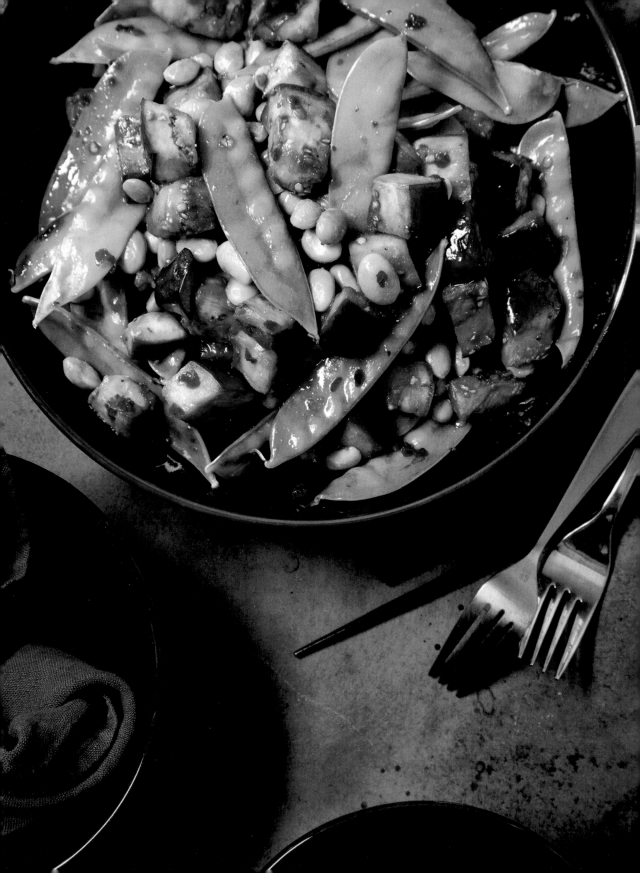

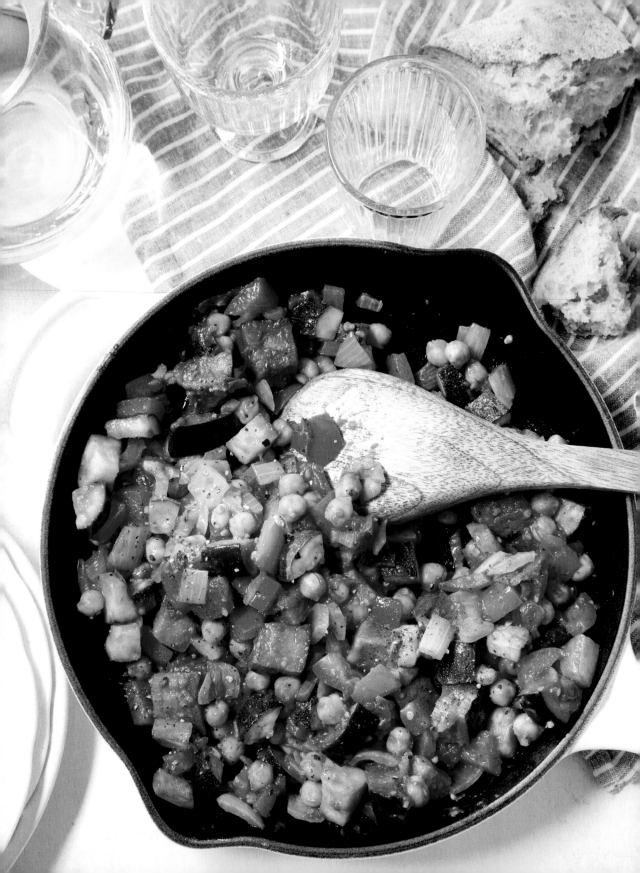

Skillet Ratatouille

I. Love. Ratatouille. Using fire-roasted canned tomatoes brings rich flavor without the long cook time. Adding chickpeas bumps up the protein!

2 cups cubed eggplant
2 cups chopped zucchini
1 cup chopped red bell pepper
1 cup chopped onion
1 teaspoon chopped garlic
⅛ teaspoon each salt and black pepper
1 cup canned garbanzo beans, drained and rinsed
½ cup canned fire-roasted diced tomatoes, lightly drained
¼ cup tomato paste
¼ teaspoon onion powder

1. Bring a skillet sprayed with nonstick spray to medium-high heat. Add eggplant and zucchini. Cook and stir until slightly softened, about 3 minutes.

2. Add bell pepper, onion, garlic, salt, and black pepper. Cook and stir until softened, about 4 minutes.

3. Add remaining ingredients. Cook and stir until hot and well mixed, about 2 minutes.

MAKES 2 SERVINGS

248 calories

Prep: 10 minutes

Cook: 10 minutes

You'll need:
skillet, nonstick spray

½ of recipe:
248 calories
2.5g total fat
(0g sat fat)
526mg sodium
49g carbs
13.5g fiber
17.5g sugars
12g protein

Stir-Frys & Skillet Meals: Meatless

So-Easy Shakshuka

230 calories

½ cup chopped bell pepper
½ cup chopped onion
One 14.5-ounce can fire-roasted diced tomatoes (not drained)
¾ cup canned cannellini (white kidney) beans, drained
    and rinsed
¼ teaspoon garlic powder
¼ teaspoon onion powder
⅛ teaspoon crushed red pepper
2 large eggs

1. Bring a skillet sprayed with nonstick spray to medium-high heat. Add bell pepper and onion. Cook and stir until mostly softened and lightly browned, about 4 minutes.

2. Add tomatoes, cannellini beans, garlic powder, onion powder, and crushed red pepper. Mix well.

3. Once simmering, reduce heat to medium. Cook and stir until slightly thickened, about 5 minutes.

4. Make 2 wells in the tomato mixture with a spoon, and crack an egg into each well. Cover and cook for 2 minutes, or until egg whites have set.

MAKES 2 SERVINGS

Prep: 5 minutes

Cook: 15 minutes

You'll need:
skillet with lid,
nonstick spray

½ of recipe:
230 calories
5g total fat
(1.5g sat fat)
695mg sodium
31g carbs
8.5g fiber
10g sugars
14g protein

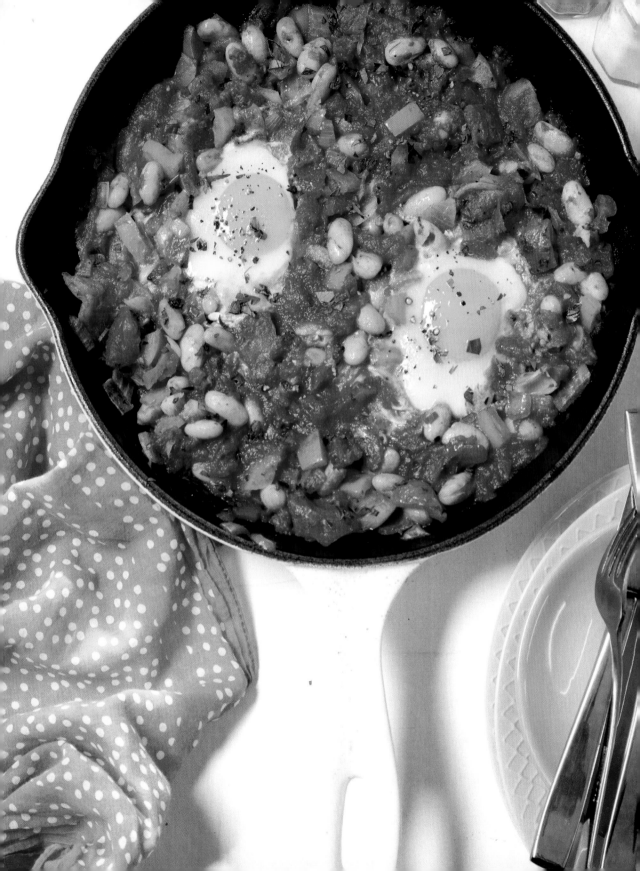

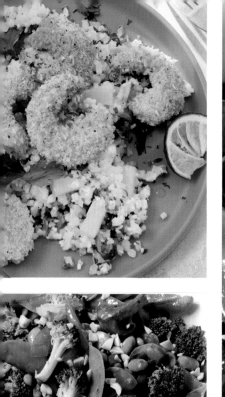
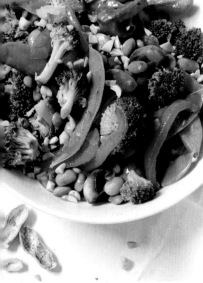
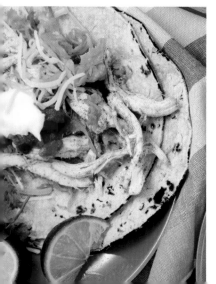
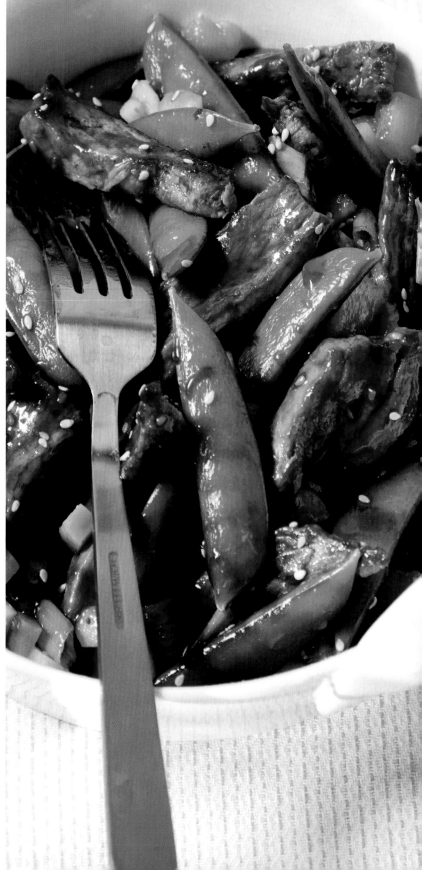

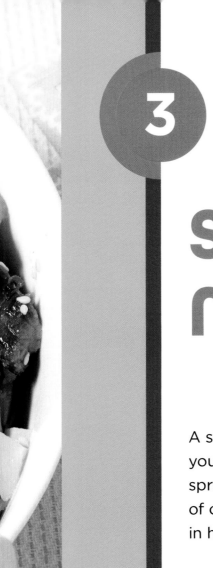

3

Sheet-Pan Meals

A simple baking sheet: the unsung hero of your kitchen. Just give it a spritz of cooking spray, load it up, and pop it in the oven. And of course, each of these recipes can be made in half an hour or less . . .

Everything Bagel Chicken

266 calories

Everything's better with everything bagel seasoning! I love how light and fresh this dish is!

5i **30m** **GF**

Prep: 5 minutes

Cook: 20 minutes

You'll need:
baking sheet,
nonstick spray

½ of recipe:
266 calories
7.5g total fat
(1g sat fat)
539mg sodium
13.5g carbs
3g fiber
7g sugars
27.5g protein

8 ounces raw boneless skinless chicken breast, cut into strips
2 cups sliced onions
2 teaspoons olive oil
1 tablespoon everything bagel seasoning
1 cup cherry tomatoes, halved

1. Preheat oven to 375 degrees. Spray a baking sheet with nonstick spray.

2. Place chicken and onions on the baking sheet. Drizzle with oil, sprinkle with seasoning, and lightly mix. Bake for 10 minutes.

3. Flip chicken and veggies, and add tomatoes to the baking sheet. Bake until chicken is fully cooked and veggies are tender, about 10 minutes.

MAKES 2 SERVINGS

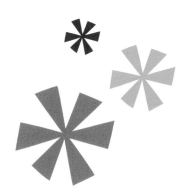

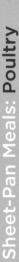

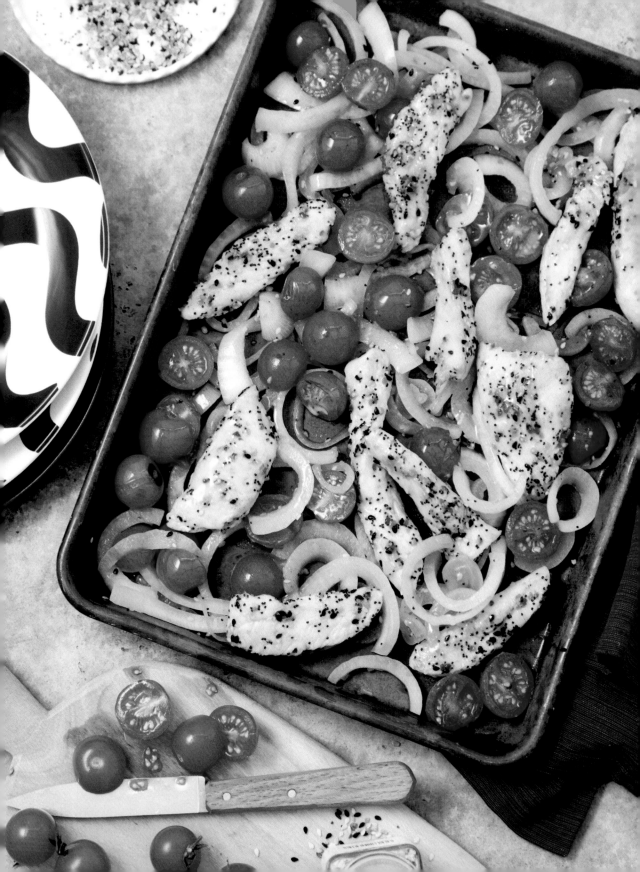

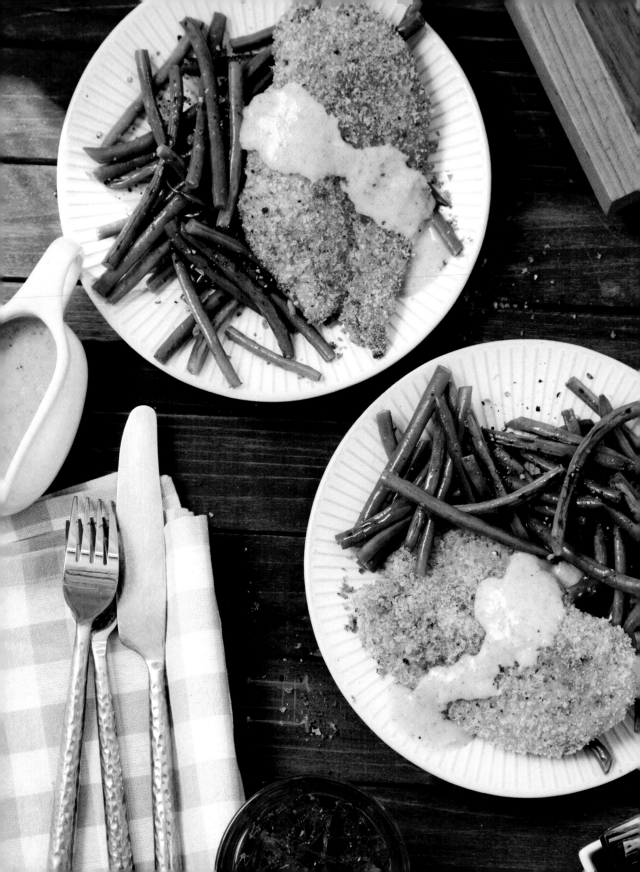

Smothered Oven-Fried Chicken Cutlets

Chicken and Veggies
½ cup panko bread crumbs
1 teaspoon garlic powder
1 teaspoon onion powder
1 teaspoon paprika
¼ teaspoon each salt and black pepper
Two 5-ounce raw boneless skinless chicken breast cutlets
2 tablespoons (about 1 large) egg white or fat-free liquid egg substitute
1 pound green beans, ends trimmed

Gravy
½ cup unsweetened plain almond milk
1 tablespoon whipped butter
1 tablespoon whole-wheat flour
⅛ teaspoon each salt and black pepper

30m

Prep: 10 minutes

Cook: 20 minutes

You'll need:
baking sheet, nonstick spray, two wide bowls, small pot, whisk

½ of recipe:
369 calories
8.5g total fat
(2.5g sat fat)
653mg sodium
33g carbs
7.5g fiber
9g sugars
40.5g protein

369 calories

1. Preheat oven to 375 degrees. Spray a baking sheet with nonstick spray.

2. In a wide bowl, combine panko, garlic powder, onion powder, paprika, and ⅛ teaspoon each salt and pepper. Mix well.

3. Place chicken in another wide bowl. Top with egg whites/substitute, and flip to coat.

4. Coat chicken with seasoned panko. Place on the baking sheet, and top with any remaining panko.

5. Add green beans to the baking sheet, and sprinkle with remaining ⅛ teaspoon each salt and pepper. Bake until chicken is cooked through and veggies are tender, about 20 minutes, flipping halfway through.

6. Meanwhile, combine gravy ingredients in a small pot. Set heat to medium low, and whisk until thickened, about 3 minutes.

7. Serve chicken topped with gravy, with green beans on the side.

MAKES 2 SERVINGS

Sheet-Pan Meals: Poultry

Sheet-Pan Tacos

323 calories

So flavorful, so easy . . . You'll want to add this into your regular rotation.

8 ounces raw boneless skinless chicken breast cutlets
1 teaspoon olive oil
1 tablespoon taco seasoning
Four 6-inch corn tortillas
½ cup shredded lettuce
2 tablespoons shredded reduced-fat Mexican-blend cheese
¼ cup salsa
2 tablespoons light sour cream
Optional topping: fresh cilantro

1. Preheat oven to 375 degrees. Spray a baking sheet with nonstick spray.

2. Place chicken on the baking sheet, drizzle with oil, and sprinkle with taco seasoning. Lightly mix. Cover with foil and bake for 20 minutes, or until cooked through.

3. Transfer chicken to a medium-large bowl, and shred with two forks.

4. Place tortillas between two damp paper towels, and microwave for 15 seconds, or until warm. Fill with lettuce, chicken, cheese, salsa, and sour cream.

MAKES 2 SERVINGS

Prep: 10 minutes

Cook: 20 minutes

You'll need:
baking sheet, nonstick spray, foil, medium-large bowl, paper towels

½ the recipe:
323 calories
9.5g total fat
(2.5g sat fat)
525mg sodium
27.5g carbs
3g fiber
4.5g sugars
30.5g protein

HG Tip
For extra flavor, char your tortillas in a dry skillet over high heat.

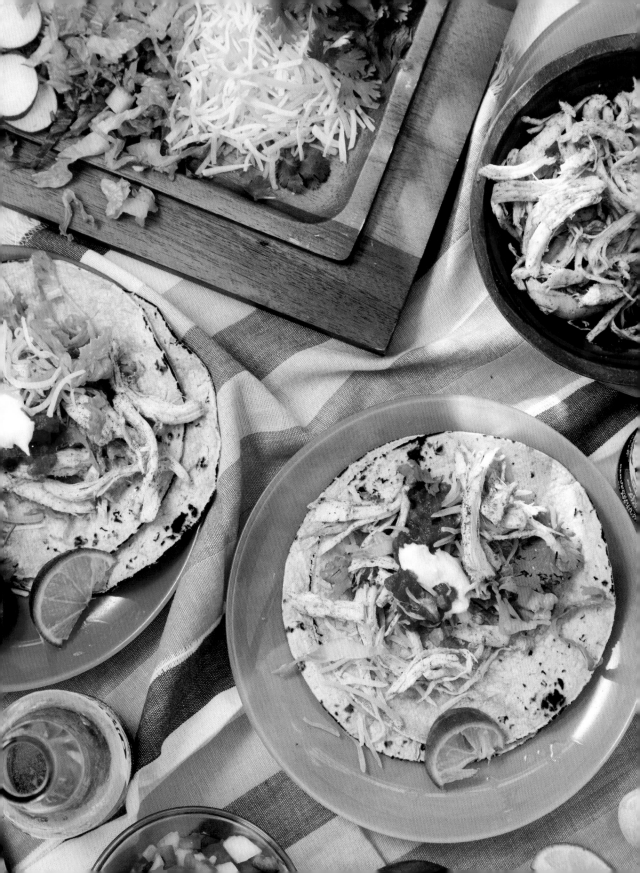

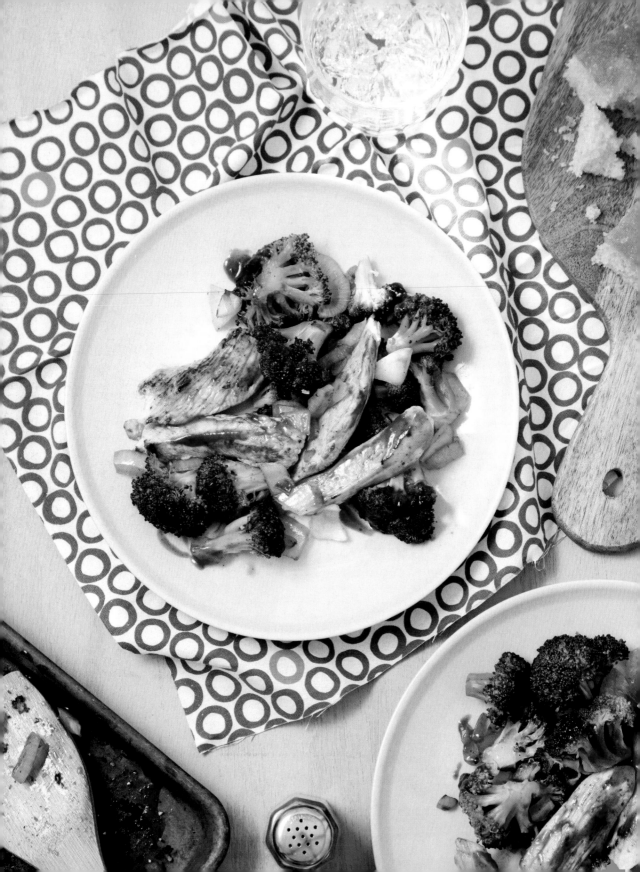

Honey BBQ Chicken & Broccoli

The combination of BBQ sauce and honey is perfection. Try it with other proteins and different veggies too!

⅓ cup BBQ sauce with 45 calories or less per 2-tablespoon serving
1½ tablespoons honey
⅛ teaspoon garlic powder
⅛ teaspoon onion powder
⅛ teaspoon each salt and black pepper
8 ounces raw boneless skinless chicken breast, cut into strips
3 cups broccoli florets
1 cup chopped onion

1. Preheat oven to 375 degrees. Spray a baking sheet with nonstick spray.

2. In a small bowl, combine BBQ sauce, honey, and seasonings. Mix well.

3. Place chicken, broccoli, and onion in a large bowl. Add sauce mixture, and toss to coat.

4. Transfer to the baking sheet. Bake until chicken is fully cooked and veggies are tender, about 20 minutes, flipping halfway through.

MAKES 2 SERVINGS

326 calories

Prep: 5 minutes

Cook: 20 minutes

You'll need:
baking sheet, nonstick spray, small bowl, large bowl

½ of recipe:
326 calories
3.5g total fat
(0.5g sat fat)
712mg sodium
44.5g carbs
4.5g fiber
29g sugars
30g protein

Sheet-Pan Meals: Poultry

Chicken Caprese

272 calories

Two 5-ounce raw boneless skinless chicken breast cutlets
¼ teaspoon each salt and black pepper
1 cup cherry tomatoes, halved
¼ cup chopped fresh basil
2 tablespoons balsamic vinegar
1 teaspoon olive oil
1 teaspoon chopped garlic
½ teaspoon Italian seasoning
⅓ cup shredded part-skim mozzarella cheese

Prep: 10 minutes

Cook: 20 minutes

You'll need:
baking sheet,
nonstick spray,
medium bowl

½ of recipe:
272 calories
9.5g total fat
(3g sat fat)
482mg sodium
6.5g carbs
1g fiber
4g sugars
37.5g protein

1. Preheat oven to 375 degrees. Spray a baking sheet with nonstick spray.

2. Place chicken on the baking sheet, and sprinkle with ⅛ teaspoon each salt and pepper. Bake for 10 minutes.

3. Meanwhile, in a medium bowl, combine tomatoes, 2 tablespoons basil, 1 tablespoon vinegar, oil, garlic, Italian seasoning, and remaining ⅛ teaspoon each salt and pepper. Toss to coat.

4. Flip chicken, and add tomatoes to the baking sheet. Bake until chicken is cooked through and tomatoes are tender, about 8 minutes.

5. Top chicken with mozzarella. Bake until melted, about 2 minutes.

6. Serve topped with remaining 2 tablespoons basil and 1 tablespoon vinegar.

MAKES 2 SERVINGS

Sheet-Pan Meals: Poultry

Hungry Girl FAST & Easy

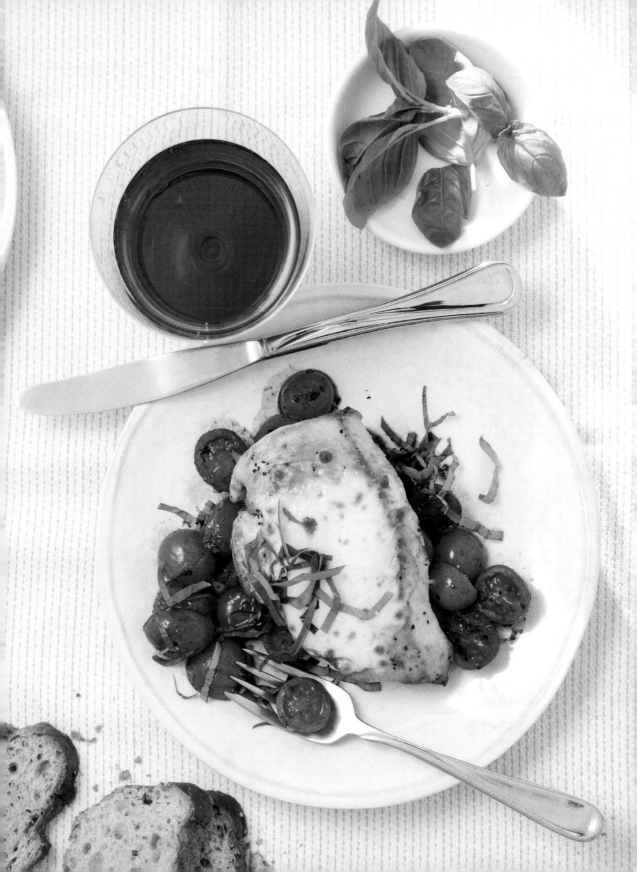

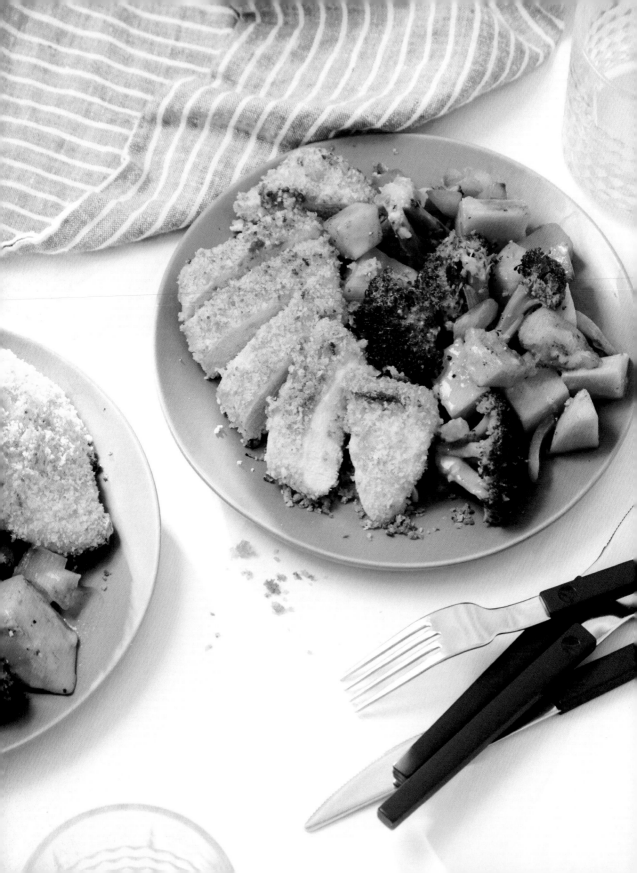

Honey Mustard Chicken

This is pure comfort food, yet it's light at the same time!

3 tablespoons Dijon mustard
1½ tablespoons honey
¼ cup panko bread crumbs
½ teaspoon garlic powder
½ teaspoon onion powder
⅛ teaspoon each salt and black pepper
Two 5-ounce raw boneless skinless chicken breast cutlets
1 cup broccoli florets
1 cup onion cut into 1-inch chunks
1 cup cubed butternut squash

1. Preheat oven to 375 degrees. Spray a baking sheet with nonstick spray.

2. In a small bowl, thoroughly mix mustard with honey.

3. In a wide bowl, mix panko with seasonings.

4. Place chicken in a second wide bowl. Add half of the honey mustard, and flip to coat. Coat chicken with seasoned panko. Place on the baking sheet, and top with any remaining panko.

5. Add broccoli and onion to the baking sheet. Bake for 10 minutes.

6. Meanwhile, place squash in a medium microwave-safe bowl. Cover and microwave for 4 minutes, or until slightly tender.

7. Flip chicken and veggies. Add squash, and top all veggies with remaining honey mustard. Bake until chicken is cooked through and veggies are tender, about 10 minutes.

MAKES 2 SERVINGS

30m

355 calories

Prep: 10 minutes

Cook: 20 minutes

You'll need:
baking sheet, nonstick spray, small bowl, two wide bowls, medium microwave-safe bowl

½ of recipe:
355 calories
4g total fat
(0.5g sat fat)
712mg sodium
39.5g carbs
4g fiber
19.5g sugars
35.5g protein

HG Tip
Look for cubed butternut squash in the produce section, or grab it from the freezer aisle. Major time-saver!

Sheet-Pan Meals: Poultry

Chicken Meatball Fajitas

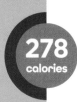

278 calories

Unconventional yet insanely delicious!

2 cups sliced bell peppers
1 cup sliced onion
1 tablespoon olive oil
1 tablespoon taco seasoning
8 ounces raw extra-lean ground chicken (at least 98% lean)
2 tablespoons (about 1 large) egg white or fat-free liquid egg substitute
2 tablespoons panko bread crumbs
¼ teaspoon each salt and black pepper
Optional topping: fresh cilantro

1. Preheat oven to 400 degrees. Spray a baking sheet with nonstick spray.

2. Place bell peppers and onion on the baking sheet. Drizzle with oil, sprinkle with 1 teaspoon taco seasoning, and lightly mix. Bake for 6 minutes.

3. Meanwhile, place chicken in a large bowl. Add remaining ingredients, including remaining 2 teaspoons taco seasoning. Mix thoroughly. Firmly form into 10 meatballs.

4. Add meatballs to the baking sheet. Bake until meatballs are cooked through and veggies are tender, 8 to 10 minutes.

MAKES 2 SERVINGS

30m

Prep: 10 minutes

Cook: 20 minutes

You'll need:
baking sheet, nonstick spray, large bowl

½ of recipe:
278 calories
9g total fat
(1g sat fat)
630mg sodium
16g carbs
3.5g fiber
6g sugars
29.5g protein

HG Tip
Can't get enough fajitas? The Steak Fajita Salad on page 43 is ready when you are . . .

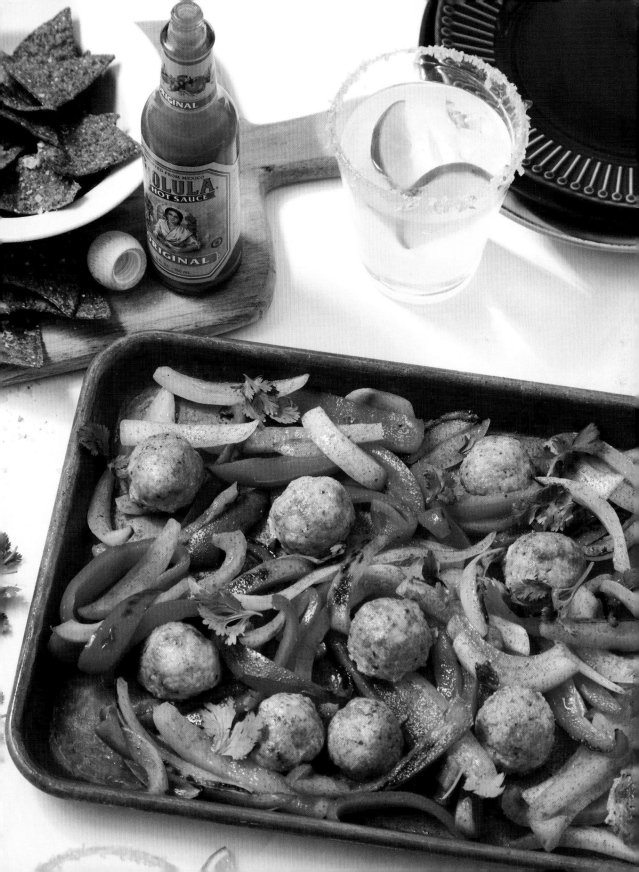

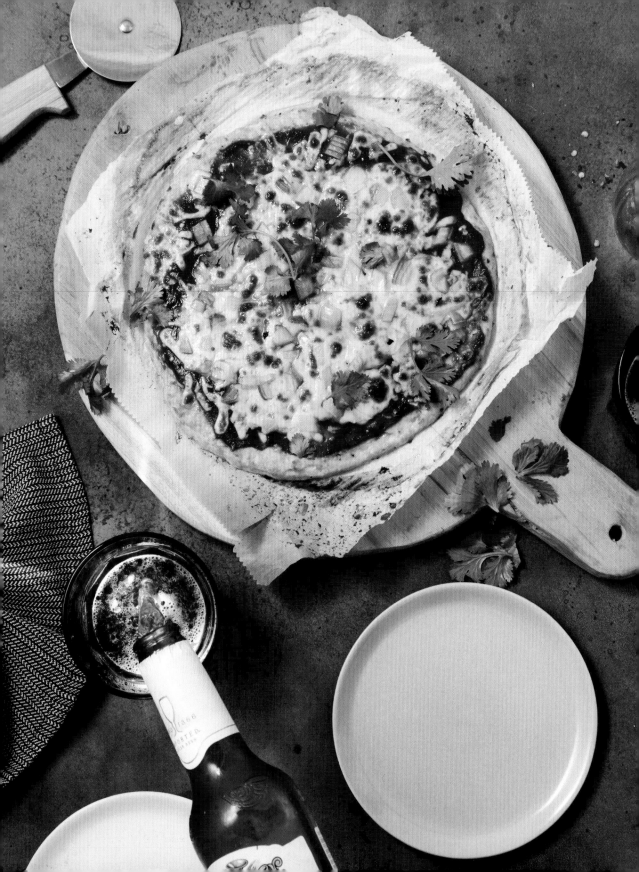

BBQ Chicken Meatza

Replacing carby pizza dough with protein-packed chicken is a really smart & delicious idea (if I do say so myself) . . .

1 pound raw extra-lean ground chicken (at least 98% lean)

2 tablespoons (about 1 large) egg white or fat-free liquid egg substitute

2 tablespoons light/reduced-fat cream cheese

1 teaspoon garlic powder

1 teaspoon onion powder

¼ teaspoon salt

⅛ teaspoon black pepper

¼ cup BBQ sauce with 45 calories or less per 2-tablespoon serving

½ cup shredded part-skim mozzarella cheese

¼ cup finely chopped red onion

2 tablespoons chopped fresh cilantro

231 calories

Prep: 10 minutes

Cook: 20 minutes

You'll need:
baking sheet, parchment paper, large bowl

¼th of recipe:
231 calories
6g total fat
(2.5g sat fat)
549mg sodium
8.5g carbs
0.5g fiber
5g sugars
31.5g protein

1. Preheat oven to 350 degrees. Line a baking sheet with parchment paper.

2. In a large bowl, combine chicken, egg white/substitute, cream cheese, and seasonings. Mix thoroughly. Shape into a circle on the baking sheet, about ¼-inch thick and 10 inches in diameter.

3. Bake until cooked through, about 15 minutes.

4. Carefully drain excess liquid, and blot dry. Spread with BBQ sauce, leaving a ½-inch border. Top with mozzarella and onion.

5. Bake until mozzarella has melted, about 5 minutes.

6. Serve topped with cilantro.

MAKES 4 SERVINGS

Sheet-Pan Meals: Poultry

BBQ Chicken Nuggets

308 calories

These nuggets are so yummy, you'll want to make 'em several times a week. Try them and see for yourself!

8 ounces raw boneless skinless chicken breast, cut into 10 nuggets

3 tablespoons BBQ sauce with 45 calories or less per 2-tablespoon serving, or more for dipping

⅓ cup panko bread crumbs

½ teaspoon garlic powder

½ teaspoon onion powder

8 ounces (about 1 medium) sweet potato, cut into 1-inch chunks

⅛ teaspoon each salt and black pepper

1. Preheat oven to 400 degrees. Spray a baking sheet with nonstick spray.

2. In a large bowl, coat chicken with BBQ sauce. In a medium bowl, combine panko, garlic powder, and onion powder, and mix well. Lightly coat chicken with seasoned panko.

3. Place chicken on the baking sheet, and top with any remaining panko. Bake for 8 minutes.

4. Meanwhile, place sweet potato in a medium microwave-safe bowl. Cover and microwave for 3 minutes, or until slightly tender.

5. Flip chicken. Add sweet potato to the baking sheet, and sprinkle with salt and pepper. Bake until chicken is fully cooked and sweet potato has lightly browned, about 8 minutes.

MAKES 2 SERVINGS

Prep: 10 minutes

Cook: 20 minutes

You'll need:
baking sheet, nonstick spray, large bowl, medium bowl, medium microwave-safe bowl

½ of recipe (5 nuggets):
308 calories
3.5g total fat
(0.5g sat fat)
550mg sodium
39g carbs
3.5g fiber
11g sugars
28.5g protein

Sheet-Pan Meals: Poultry

Hungry Girl *FAST & Easy*

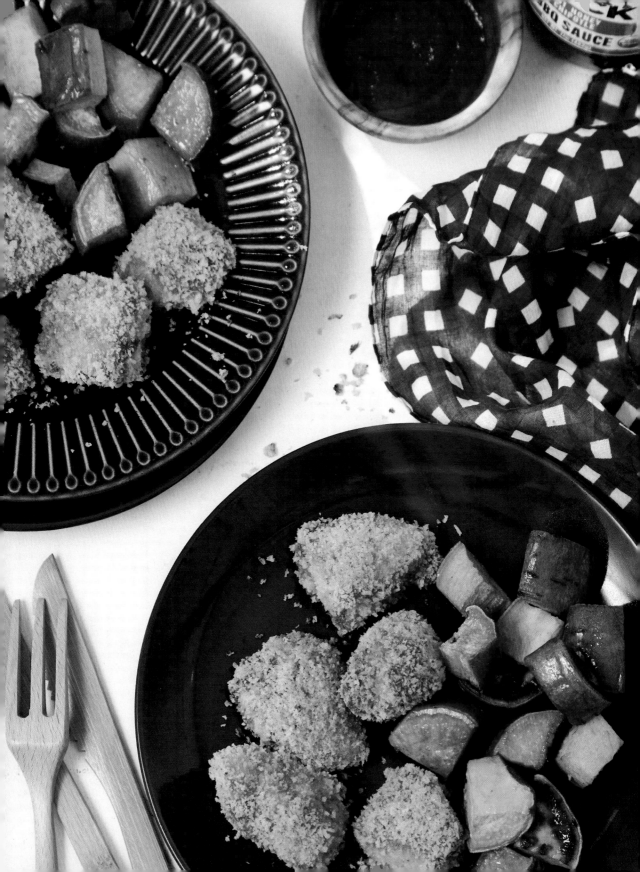

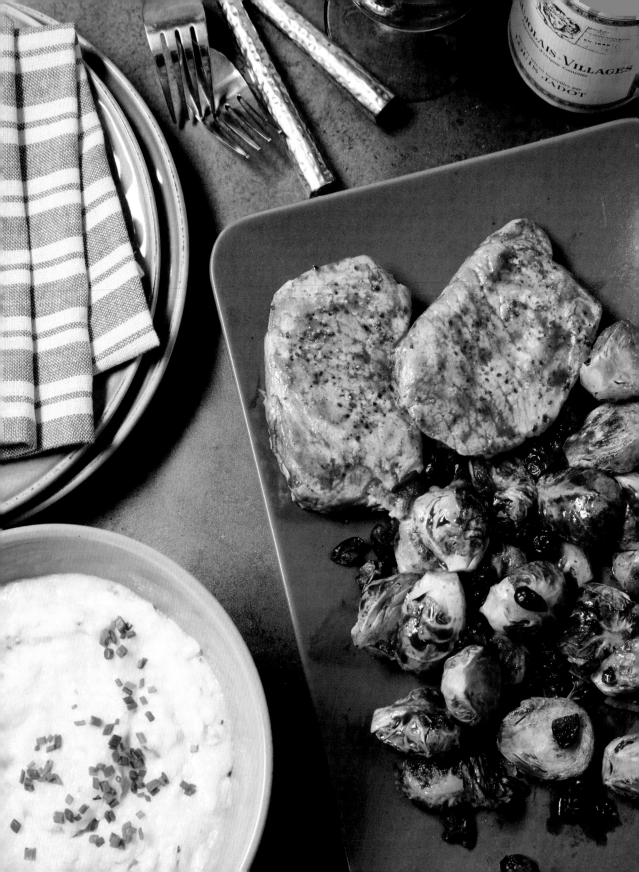

Cranberry Balsamic Pork Chops

Sheet-pan pork chops are SO tender. This is a great dish for fall (or anytime, really)!

¼ cup balsamic vinegar
1½ teaspoons olive oil
1½ teaspoons Dijon mustard
Two 4-ounce raw boneless pork chops (about ½-inch thick)
¼ teaspoon each salt and black pepper
8 ounces (about 16 medium) Brussels sprouts, trimmed and halved
2 tablespoons sweetened dried cranberries, chopped

1. Preheat oven to 400 degrees. Spray a baking sheet with nonstick spray.

2. In a small bowl, combine vinegar, oil, and mustard. Mix well.

3. Place pork chops on the baking sheet, and sprinkle with ⅛ teaspoon each salt and pepper. Bake for 10 minutes.

4. Meanwhile, place Brussels sprouts in a medium microwave-safe bowl with ¼ cup water. Cover and microwave for 4 minutes, or until softened. Drain excess liquid.

5. Add Brussels sprouts to the baking sheet, and sprinkle with remaining ⅛ teaspoon each salt and pepper. Drizzle pork and Brussels sprouts with vinegar mixture, and top with cranberries. Bake until pork is cooked through and veggies are tender, about 5 minutes.

MAKES 2 SERVINGS

30m **GF**

306 calories

Prep: 5 minutes

Cook: 15 minutes

You'll need:
baking sheet, nonstick spray, small bowl, medium microwave-safe bowl

½ of recipe:
306 calories
11.5g total fat
(3g sat fat)
452mg sodium
21.5g carbs
4.5g fiber
12g sugars
28g protein

Sheet-Pan Meals: **Beef & Pork**

Pineapple BBQ Pork Chops

332 calories

½ cup canned crushed pineapple packed in juice (not drained)

¼ cup BBQ sauce with about 45 calories or less per 2-tablespoon serving

Two 4-ounce raw boneless pork chops (about ½-inch thick)

¼ teaspoon each salt and black pepper

2 cups broccoli florets

1 cup roughly chopped onion

1 cup cherry tomatoes, halved

Optional: chopped fresh cilantro

Prep: 10 minutes

Cook: 15 minutes

You'll need:
baking sheet, nonstick spray, medium bowl

½ of recipe:
332 calories
8.5g total fat
(3g sat fat)
736mg sodium
35.5g carbs
5g fiber
22.5g sugars
28.5g protein

1. Preheat oven to 400 degrees. Spray a baking sheet with nonstick spray.

2. In a medium bowl, mix pineapple with BBQ sauce.

3. Season pork chops with ⅛ teaspoon each salt and pepper, and place on the baking sheet. Add broccoli and onion, and sprinkle with remaining ⅛ teaspoon each salt and pepper. Bake for 10 minutes.

4. Flip pork chops and veggies. Top with sauce mixture, and add tomatoes to the baking sheet. Bake until pork is cooked through and veggies are tender, about 5 minutes.

MAKES 2 SERVINGS

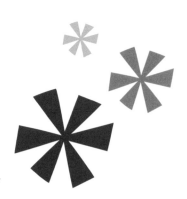

Sheet-Pan Meals: Beef & Pork

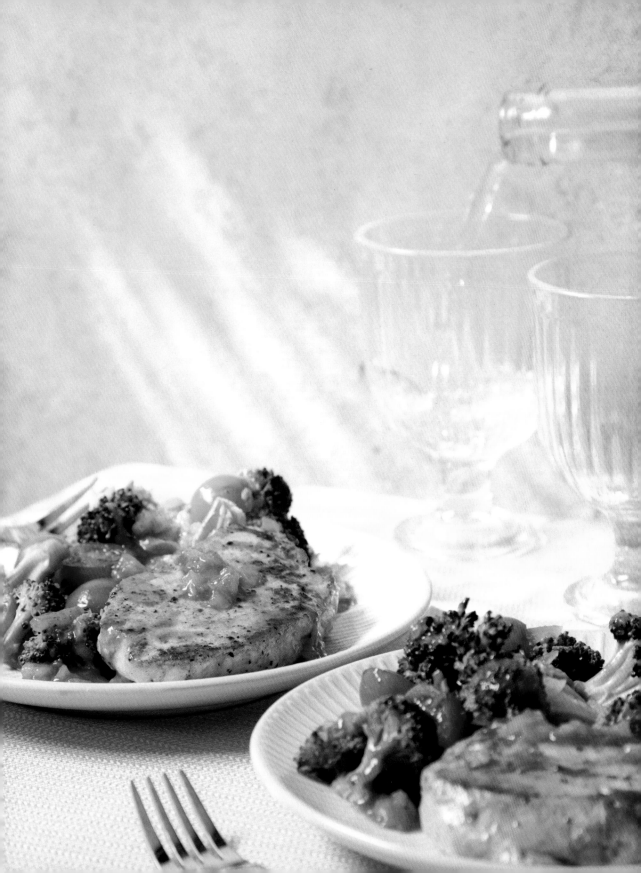

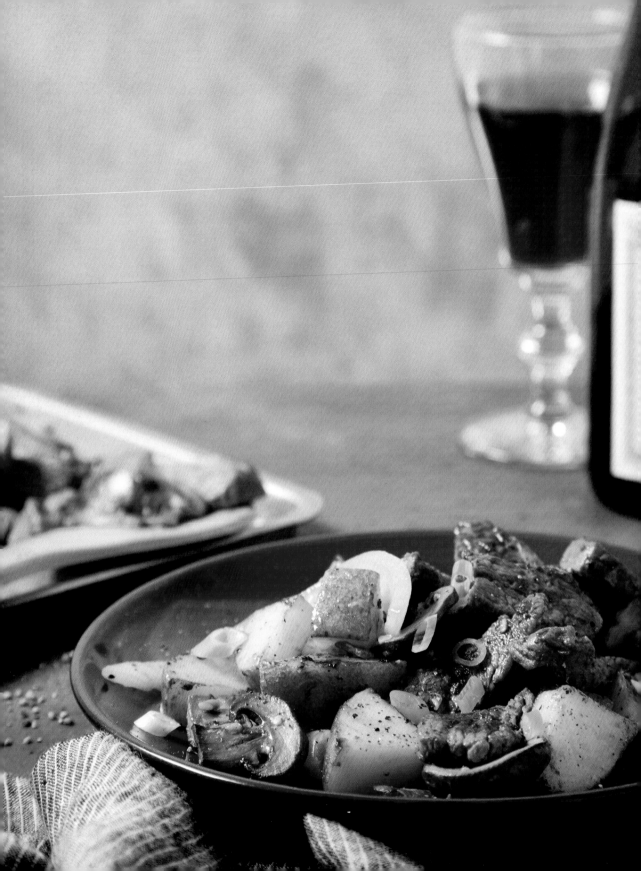

Garlic Steak & Potatoes

A full steak dinner, ready in 30! Fair warning: If you serve this to a date, expect a marriage proposal by the end of the night.

 30m **GF**

316 calories

Prep: 10 minutes

Cook: 20 minutes

You'll need: baking sheet, nonstick spray, medium microwave-safe bowl

½ of recipe:
316 calories
11.5g total fat
(3.5g sat fat)
670mg sodium
24g carbs
3g fiber
5g sugars
29g protein

2 cups sliced brown mushrooms
1 cup sliced onion
6 ounces (about 3) baby red potatoes, cut into ½-inch chunks
8 ounces thinly sliced raw lean flank steak
1 tablespoon chopped garlic
2 teaspoons olive oil
½ teaspoon salt
¼ teaspoon black pepper
¼ teaspoon garlic powder
¼ teaspoon onion powder
2 tablespoons chopped scallions

1. Preheat oven to 400 degrees. Spray a baking sheet with nonstick spray.

2. Add mushrooms and onion to the baking sheet, and bake for 12 minutes.

3. Meanwhile, place potatoes in a medium microwave-safe bowl. Cover and microwave for 3 minutes, or until slightly tender.

4. Flip veggies, and add potatoes and steak to the baking sheet. Sprinkle with chopped garlic, oil, and seasonings. Lightly stir.

5. Bake until steak is fully cooked and potatoes and veggies are tender, about 8 minutes.

6. Serve topped with scallions.

MAKES 2 SERVINGS

Sheet-Pan Meals: **Beef & Pork**

Teriyaki Beef

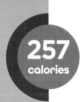

257 calories

2 tablespoons thick teriyaki sauce or marinade
1 tablespoon orange juice
8 ounces thinly sliced raw lean flank steak
2 cups sugar snap peas
¼ teaspoon garlic powder
⅛ teaspoon ground ginger
Dash each salt and black pepper
½ cup canned sliced water chestnuts, drained and chopped
¼ cup chopped scallions

1. Preheat oven to 400 degrees. Spray a baking sheet with nonstick spray.

2. In a small bowl, mix teriyaki with orange juice.

3. Place steak and sugar snap peas on the baking sheet, and sprinkle with seasonings. Bake for 8 minutes.

4. Flip steak and sugar snap peas. Add water chestnuts and scallions, and drizzle with sauce mixture. Bake until steak is cooked through and veggies are tender, about 2 minutes.

MAKES 2 SERVINGS

 30m

Prep: 10 minutes

Cook: 10 minutes

You'll need:
baking sheet,
nonstick spray,
small bowl

½ of recipe:
257 calories
7.5g total fat
(3g sat fat)
580mg sodium
19.5g carbs
4g fiber
8.5g sugars
27.5g protein

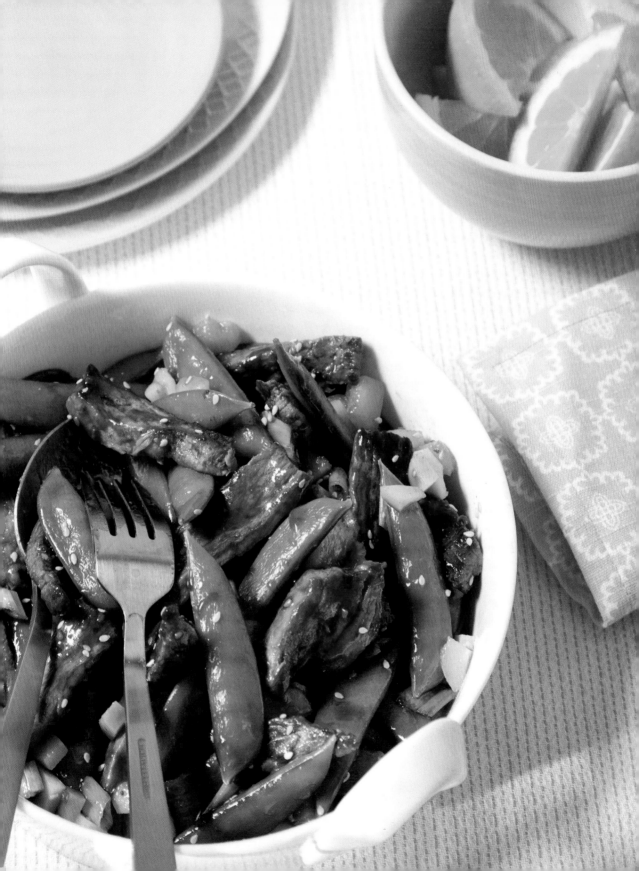

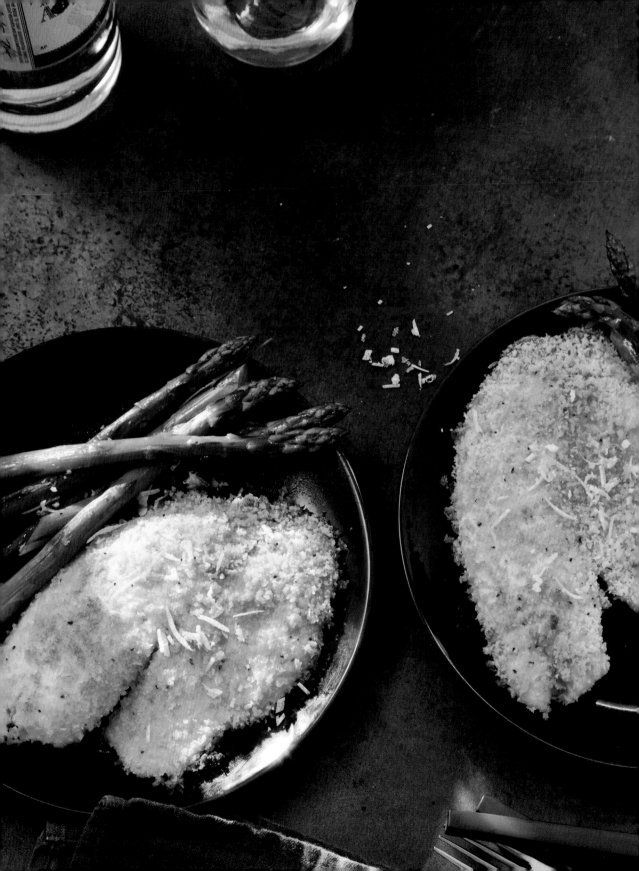

Crispy Lemon Parm Tilapia

The lemon zest brings so much flavor to the table! Feel free to make this one with any fish you like . . .

 30m

Prep: 10 minutes

Cook: 15 minutes

You'll need:
grater/zester, baking sheet, nonstick spray, two wide bowls

½ of recipe:
261 calories
6g total fat
(2.5g sat fat)
430mg sodium
12.5g carbs
3g fiber
3.5g sugars
41g protein

261 calories

¼ cup panko bread crumbs
2 tablespoons plus 2 teaspoons grated Parmesan cheese
¾ teaspoon garlic powder
Dash each salt and black pepper
¼ cup (about 2 large) egg whites or fat-free liquid egg substitute
2 tablespoons lemon juice
Two 5-ounce raw tilapia fillets
12 asparagus spears, tough ends removed
1 teaspoon lemon zest

1. Preheat oven to 400 degrees. Spray a baking sheet with nonstick spray.

2. In a wide bowl, combine panko, 2 tablespoons Parm, ½ teaspoon garlic powder, salt, and pepper. Mix well.

3. In another wide bowl, mix egg whites/substitute with lemon juice. Add tilapia, and flip to coat.

4. Coat tilapia with seasoned panko. Place on the baking sheet, and top with any remaining panko. Add asparagus, and sprinkle with remaining ¼ teaspoon garlic powder and 2 teaspoons Parm.

5. Bake until fish is cooked through, coating is crispy, and asparagus is tender, about 12 minutes, flipping halfway through.

6. Serve topped with lemon zest.

MAKES 2 SERVINGS

HG FYI
One lemon is all you'll need for this recipe . . . That'll give you plenty of juice and zest!

Sheet-Pan Meals: Seafood

Tropical Coconut Shrimp

296 calories

This seafood dish is a crowd pleaser! And just 20 minutes, start to finish . . .

⅓ cup panko bread crumbs

¼ cup unsweetened shredded coconut

1 teaspoon garlic powder

¼ teaspoon each salt and black pepper

¼ cup (about 2 large) egg whites or fat-free liquid egg substitute

½ teaspoon coconut extract

8 ounces (about 16) raw large shrimp, peeled, tails removed, deveined

2½ cups frozen riced cauliflower

⅓ cup pineapple tidbits packed in juice, drained

2 tablespoons chopped cilantro, or more for topping

2 tablespoons finely chopped red onion

Optional topping: sweet chili sauce

1. Preheat oven to 400 degrees. Spray a baking sheet with nonstick spray.

2. In a wide bowl, combine panko, shredded coconut, garlic powder, and ⅛ teaspoon each salt and pepper. Mix well.

3. In another wide bowl, mix egg whites/substitute with ¼ teaspoon coconut extract. Add shrimp, and flip to coat.

4. Coat shrimp with panko mixture. Place on the baking sheet, and top with any remaining panko. Bake until cooked through and crispy, about 4 minutes per side.

5. Meanwhile, place cauliflower in a medium-large microwave-safe bowl. Microwave for 2 minutes, or until hot. Add pineapple, cilantro, onion, remaining ¼ teaspoon coconut extract, and remaining ⅛ teaspoon each salt and pepper. Mix well. Microwave until hot, about 1 minute.

6. Serve shrimp with cauliflower rice.

MAKES 2 SERVINGS

30m

Prep: 10 minutes

Cook: 10 minutes

You'll need: baking sheet, nonstick spray, two wide bowls, medium-large microwave-safe bowl

½ of recipe:
296 calories
7.5g total fat
(5.5g sat fat)
766mg sodium
26.5g carbs
5.5g fiber
10g sugars
29.5g protein

HG FYI
Frozen riced cauliflower is a time-saving staple! If you'd rather DIY, flip to page 312 for the 411.

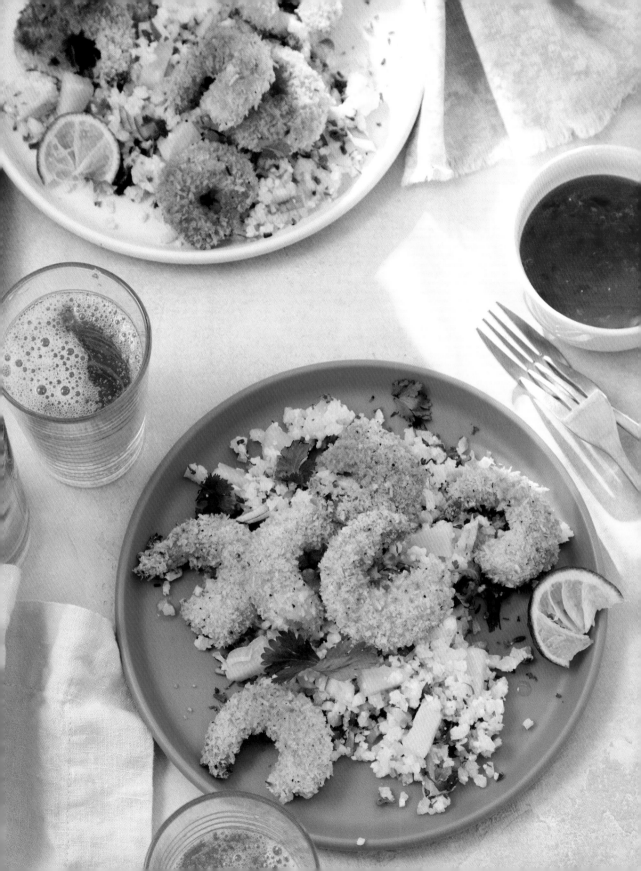

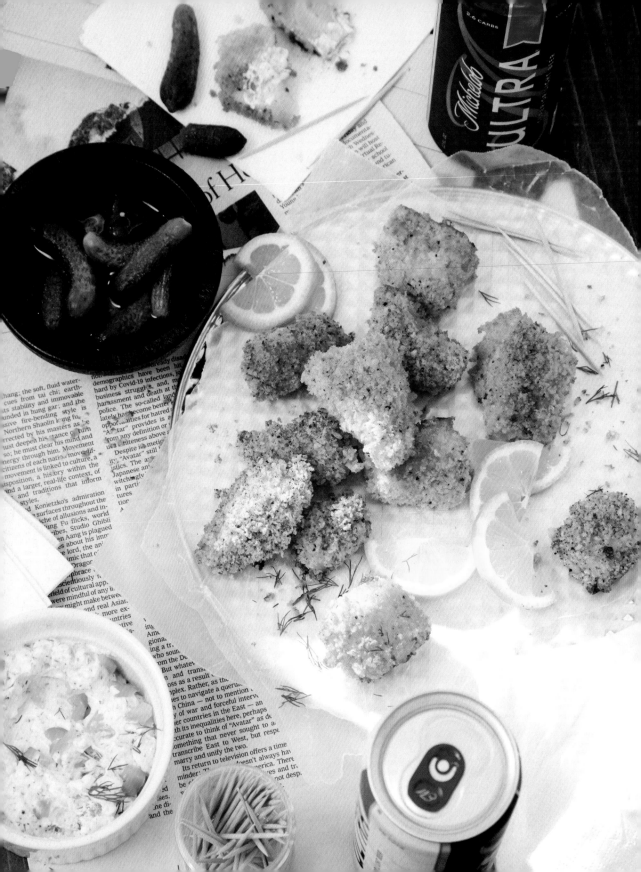

Oven-Fried Fish Nuggets

These are next-level fish sticks! You'll want to dip EVERYTHING in the easy homemade tartar sauce.

⅓ cup panko bread crumbs
½ teaspoon chili powder
½ teaspoon plus dash garlic powder
¼ teaspoon each salt and black pepper
8 ounces raw cod fillet, cut into 10 nuggets
¼ cup (about 2 large) egg whites or fat-free liquid egg substitute
2 tablespoons light mayonnaise
1 tablespoon light/reduced-fat cream cheese
1 tablespoon fat-free plain Greek yogurt
1 tablespoon chopped dill pickles
¼ teaspoon dried dill

1. Preheat oven to 400 degrees. Spray a baking sheet with nonstick spray.

2. In a wide bowl, mix panko with chili powder, ½ teaspoon garlic powder, salt, and pepper.

3. Place cod in another wide bowl. Add egg whites/substitute, and flip to coat.

4. Coat cod with seasoned panko. Place on the baking sheet, and top with any remaining panko. Bake until fully cooked and crispy, about 5 minutes per side.

5. In a small bowl, combine mayo, cream cheese, yogurt, pickles, dill, and remaining dash garlic powder. Mix well, and serve with fish nuggets for dipping.

MAKES 2 SERVINGS

 30m

Prep: 10 minutes

Cook: 10 minutes

218 calories

You'll need:
baking sheet, nonstick spray, two wide bowls, small bowl

½ of recipe:
218 calories
6.5g total fat
(1.5g sat fat)
651mg sodium
11.5g carbs
0.5g fiber
1.5g sugars
26g protein

Sheet-Pan Meals: Seafood

Caribbean Salmon

336 calories

Send your mouth on a tropical vacation! The pineapple and cilantro play so well together here . . .

Two 4-ounce raw skinless salmon fillets
¼ teaspoon chili powder
¼ teaspoon garlic powder
¼ teaspoon onion powder
¼ teaspoon plus ⅛ teaspoon each salt and black pepper
1 pound green beans, ends trimmed
2 teaspoons olive oil
½ cup pineapple tidbits packed in juice, drained
½ cup chopped tomato
2 tablespoons chopped cilantro

1. Preheat oven to 375 degrees. Spray a baking sheet with nonstick spray.

2. Place salmon on the baking sheet, and sprinkle with chili powder, garlic powder, onion powder, and ⅛ teaspoon each salt and pepper.

3. Add green beans to the baking sheet, drizzle with oil, and sprinkle with ⅛ teaspoon salt and pepper. Lightly mix.

4. Bake until salmon is cooked through and green beans are tender, about 14 minutes, flipping veggies halfway through.

5. In a medium bowl, combine pineapple, tomato, cilantro, and remaining ⅛ teaspoon each salt and pepper. Mix well. Serve over salmon, with green beans on the side.

MAKES 2 SERVINGS

Prep: 10 minutes

Cook: 15 minutes

You'll need:
baking sheet, nonstick spray, medium bowl

½ of recipe:
336 calories
14.5g total fat
(3g sat fat)
539mg sodium
26g carbs
7.5g fiber
15.5g sugars
28g protein

Sheet-Pan Meals: Seafood

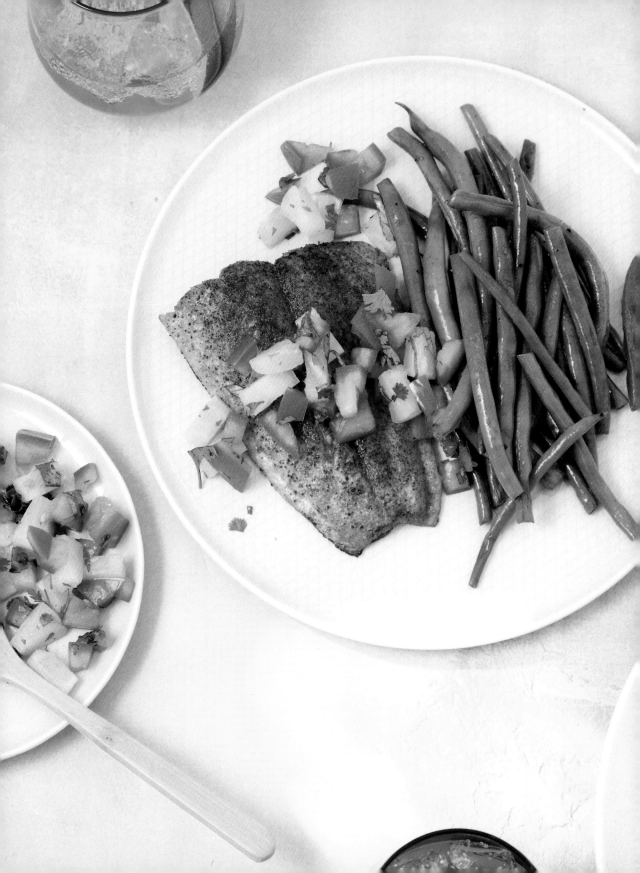

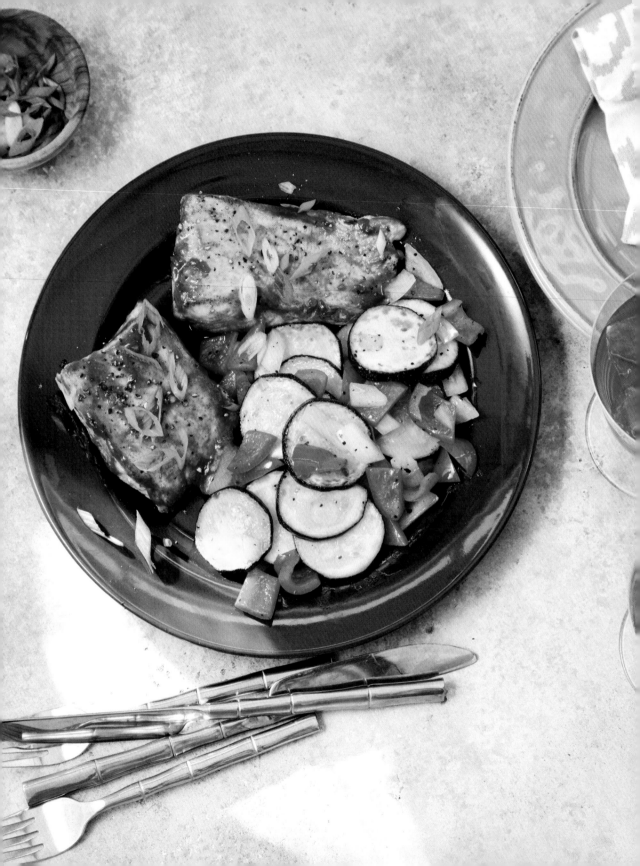

A sweet & tangy sheet-pan superstar! This may be my favorite salmon recipe in the book. (Shhhh . . . Don't tell the others.)

 30m **GF**

Prep: 10 minutes

Cook: 15 minutes

308 calories

2 tablespoons BBQ sauce with 45 calories or less per 2-tablespoon serving
1 tablespoon sweet chili sauce
Two 4-ounce raw skinless salmon fillets
¼ teaspoon garlic powder
¼ teaspoon onion powder
¼ teaspoon each salt and black pepper
1½ cups zucchini sliced into coins
½ cup roughly chopped red bell peppers
½ cup roughly chopped onion
2 teaspoons olive oil
Optional topping: scallions

You'll need:
baking sheet, nonstick spray, small bowl

½ of recipe:
308 calories
14g total fat
(3g sat fat)
676mg sodium
19.5g carbs
2.5g fiber
13.5g sugars
25.5g protein

1. Preheat oven to 375 degrees. Spray a baking sheet with nonstick spray.

2. In a small bowl, mix BBQ sauce with chili sauce.

3. Place salmon on the baking sheet, and season with garlic powder, onion powder, and ⅛ teaspoon each salt and black pepper.

4. Add veggies to the baking sheet, drizzle with oil, and sprinkle with remaining ⅛ teaspoon each salt and black pepper. Lightly mix. Bake for 7 minutes.

5. Flip veggies, and spoon sauce over salmon. Bake until salmon is cooked through and veggies are tender, about 7 minutes.

MAKES 2 SERVINGS

Sheet-Pan Meals: Seafood

Coconut-Crusted Cod

Another flavor-packed home run. Serve it up over steamed veggies, riced cauliflower, or even a big green salad.

¼ cup panko bread crumbs

3 tablespoons unsweetened shredded coconut

½ teaspoon chili powder

½ teaspoon garlic powder

¼ teaspoon each salt and black pepper

¼ cup (about 2 large) egg whites or fat-free liquid egg substitute

¼ teaspoon coconut extract

Two 5-ounce raw cod fillets

2 tablespoons sweet chili sauce

1. Preheat oven to 400 degrees. Spray a baking sheet with nonstick spray.

2. In a wide bowl, combine panko, shredded coconut, and seasonings. Mix well.

3. In another wide bowl, mix egg whites/substitute with coconut extract. Add cod, and flip to coat.

4. Coat cod with seasoned panko. Place on the baking sheet, and top with any remaining panko.

5. Bake until fish is cooked through and coating is crispy, about 6 minutes per side.

6. Serve drizzled with chili sauce.

MAKES 2 SERVINGS

Prep: 5 minutes

Cook: 15 minutes

You'll need:
baking sheet, nonstick spray, two wide bowls

½ of recipe:
253 calories
5.5g total fat
(4g sat fat)
698mg sodium
18.5g carbs
1.5g fiber
9g sugars
30g protein

HG Tip
Crisp up your leftovers in an air fryer!

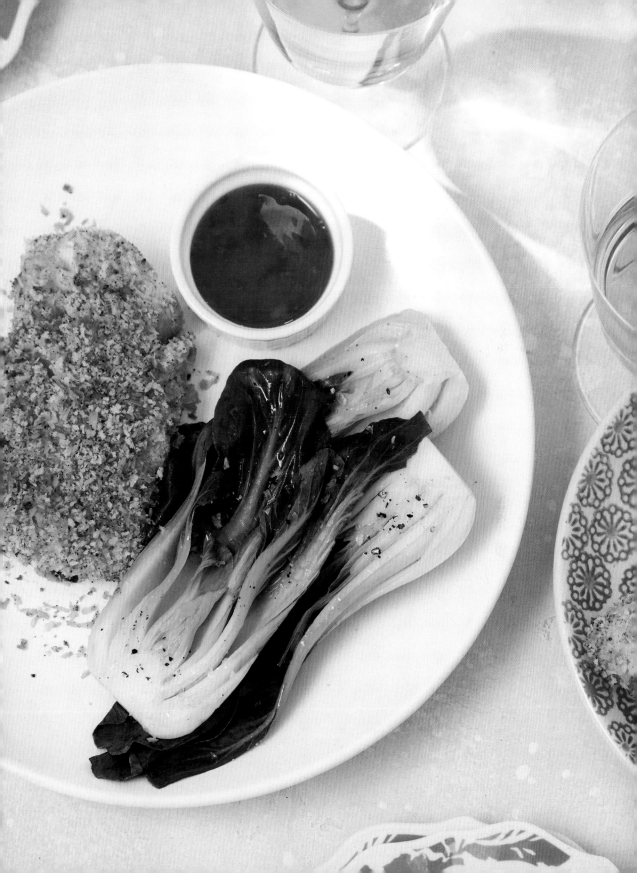

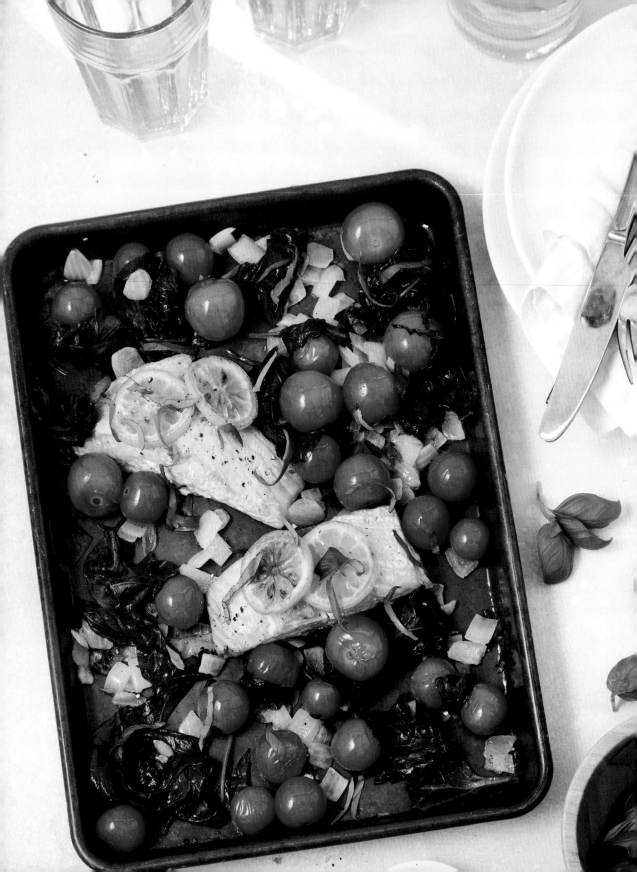

Lemon Basil Salmon

Two 4-ounce raw skinless salmon fillets
¼ teaspoon each salt and black pepper
4 slices lemon
2 cups cherry tomatoes
1 cup chopped onion
2 teaspoons olive oil
4 cups spinach
2 tablespoons chopped fresh basil

1. Preheat oven to 375 degrees. Spray a baking sheet with nonstick spray.

2. Place salmon on the baking sheet, and sprinkle with ⅛ teaspoon each salt and pepper. Top with lemon.

3. Add tomatoes and onion to the baking sheet. Drizzle with oil, and sprinkle with remaining ⅛ teaspoon each salt and pepper. Lightly mix.

4. Bake until salmon is cooked through and tomatoes have softened, about 14 minutes, flipping veggies halfway through.

5. Add spinach and basil, and bake until wilted, about 2 minutes.

MAKES 2 SERVINGS

305 calories

Prep: 5 minutes

Cook: 20 minutes

You'll need:
baking sheet,
nonstick spray

½ of recipe:
305 calories
14.5g total fat
(3g sat fat)
426mg sodium
17.5g carbs
5g fiber
8g sugars
27.5g protein

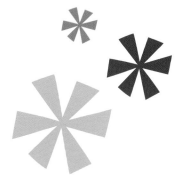

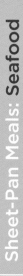
Sheet-Pan Meals: Seafood

Mustard-Crusted Salmon

321 calories

¼ cup panko bread crumbs
½ teaspoon garlic powder
½ teaspoon onion powder
¼ teaspoon each salt and black pepper
Two 4-ounce raw skinless salmon fillets
2 tablespoons whole-grain mustard
2 cups broccoli florets
12 asparagus spears, tough ends removed
2 teaspoons olive oil

1. Preheat oven to 375 degrees. Spray a baking sheet with nonstick spray.

2. In a small bowl, combine panko, garlic powder, onion powder, and ⅛ teaspoon each salt and pepper. Mix well.

3. Place salmon on the baking sheet, and spread with mustard. Top with seasoned panko.

4. Add broccoli and asparagus to the baking sheet, drizzle with oil, and sprinkle with remaining ⅛ teaspoon each salt and pepper. Lightly mix.

5. Bake until salmon is cooked through and veggies are tender, about 14 minutes, flipping veggies halfway through.

MAKES 2 SERVINGS

30m

Prep: 10 minutes

Cook: 15 minutes

You'll need:
baking sheet,
nonstick spray,
small bowl

½ of recipe:
321 calories
14.5g total fat
(3g sat fat)
606mg sodium
17.5g carbs
5g fiber
4.5g sugars
29.5g protein

Sheet-Pan Meals: Seafood

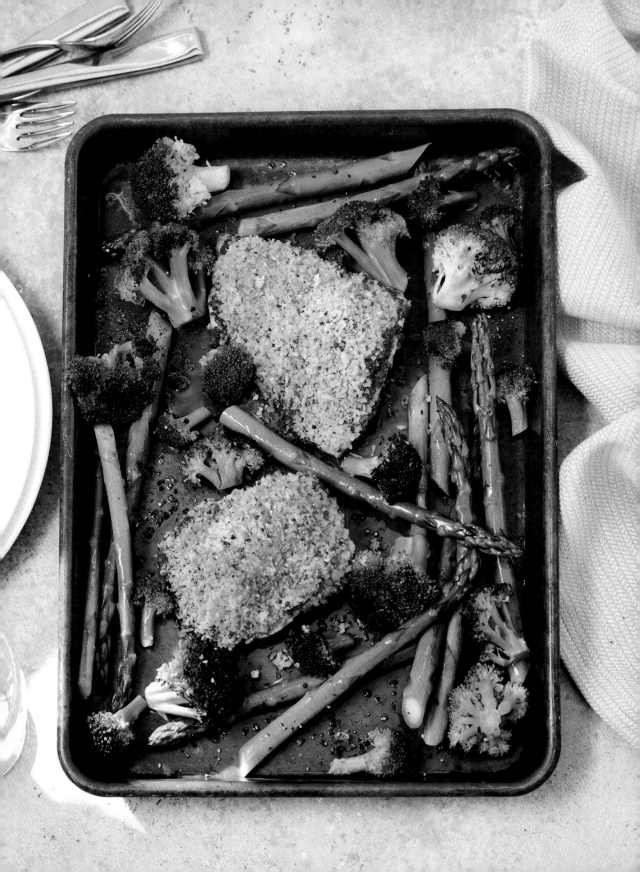

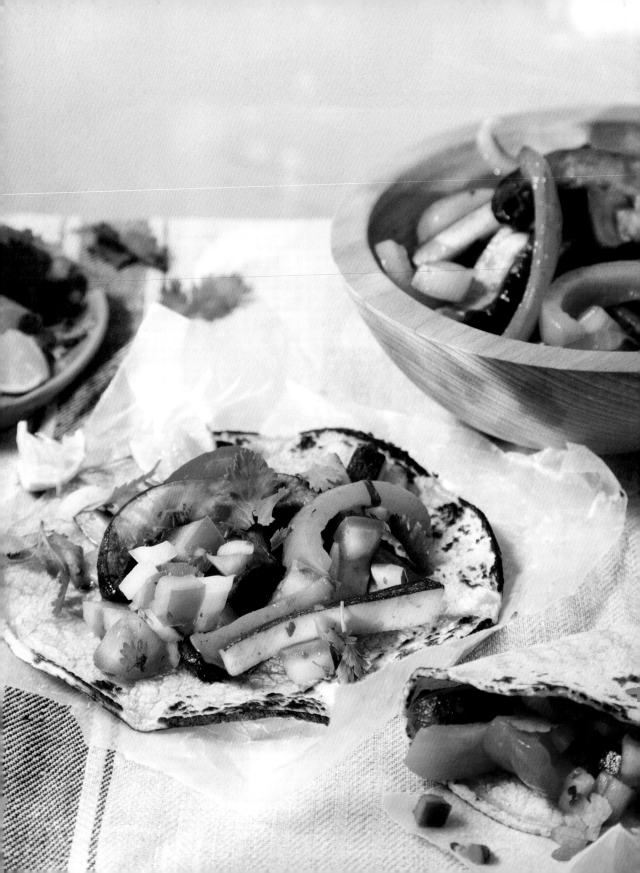

Fajita-Style Veggie Tacos

2 large portabella mushrooms, sliced
1 cup sliced bell pepper
1 cup sliced onion
1 cup zucchini cut into strips
1 tablespoon olive oil
2 teaspoons lime juice
1 tablespoon taco seasoning
¼ teaspoon salt
Four 6-inch corn tortillas
2 tablespoons chopped fresh cilantro
Optional topping: salsa

1. Preheat oven to 400 degrees. Spray a baking sheet with nonstick spray.

2. Place veggies on the baking sheet. Drizzle with oil and lime juice, and sprinkle with taco seasoning and salt. Lightly mix.

3. Bake until tender, about 20 minutes, flipping halfway through.

4. Place tortillas between two damp paper towels, and microwave for 15 seconds, or until warm. Fill with veggies and cilantro.

MAKES 2 SERVINGS

Prep: 10 minutes

Cook: 20 minutes

You'll need:
baking sheet,
nonstick spray,
paper towels

½ of recipe:
253 calories
9g total fat
(1g sat fat)
535mg sodium
39.5g carbs
7g fiber
9g sugars
7g protein

253 calories

Sheet-Pan Meals: Meatless

Sweet Teriyaki Tofu

252 calories

8 ounces block-style extra-firm tofu, excess moisture removed, cut into 1-inch cubes
½ teaspoon garlic powder
⅛ teaspoon each salt and black pepper
4 cups broccoli florets
2 tablespoons thick teriyaki sauce or marinade
1 tablespoon sweet chili sauce
1 teaspoon sesame oil
¼ cup chopped scallions

1. Preheat oven to 400 degrees. Spray a baking sheet with nonstick spray.

2. Season tofu with garlic powder, salt, and pepper, and place on the baking sheet. Add broccoli, and bake until tofu is crisp and broccoli is tender, about 20 minutes, flipping halfway through.

3. In a small bowl, mix teriyaki, chili sauce, and oil. Drizzle over tofu and broccoli, and toss to mix.

4. Serve topped with scallions.

MAKES 2 SERVINGS

Prep: 5 minutes

Cook: 20 minutes

You'll need:
baking sheet, nonstick spray, small bowl

½ of recipe:
252 calories
9.5g total fat
(1g sat fat)
750mg sodium
25.5g carbs
6g fiber
11g sugars
18.5g protein

HG Tip
Find sweet chili sauce with the shelf-stable Asian ingredients. It's a great pantry staple!

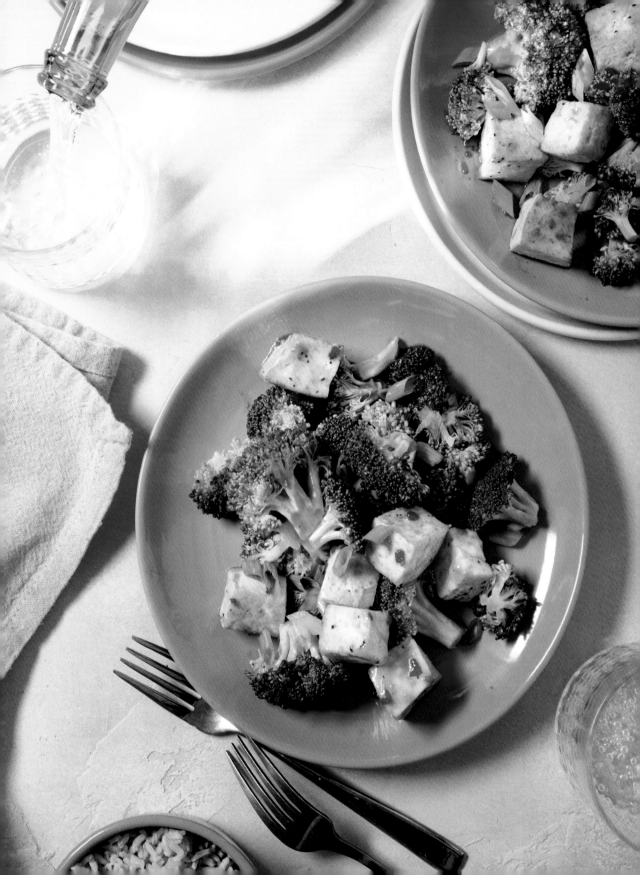

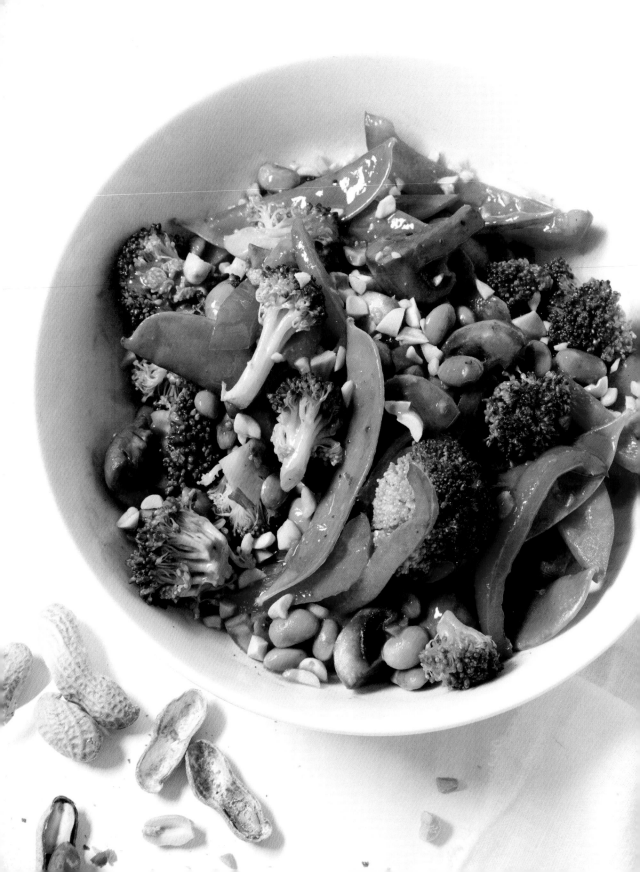

Thai Peanut Veggies

2 cups broccoli florets
1½ cups quartered mushrooms
1 cup sliced red bell pepper
1 cup snow peas
½ cup frozen shelled edamame
2 teaspoons olive oil
¼ teaspoon each salt and black pepper
¼ cup Thai peanut sauce/salad dressing with 65 calories or less per 2-tablespoon serving
¼ ounce (about 1 tablespoon) chopped roasted unsalted peanuts

Prep: 10 minutes

Cook: 20 minutes

You'll need:
baking sheet, nonstick spray

½ of recipe:
247 calories
12g total fat
(1.5g sat fat)
649mg sodium
25.5g carbs
7.5g fiber
13g sugars
12.5g protein

1. Preheat oven to 400 degrees. Spray a baking sheet with nonstick spray.

2. Place veggies on the baking sheet. Drizzle with oil, and sprinkle with salt and black pepper. Lightly mix.

3. Bake until tender, about 20 minutes, flipping halfway through.

4. Drizzle with peanut sauce/dressing, and toss to mix.

5. Serve topped with peanuts.

MAKES 2 SERVINGS

HG FYI
Whole Foods 365 Everyday Value makes an excellent Thai peanut sauce. (You can also DIY with the recipe on page 265!)

Sheet-Pan Meals: Meatless

Crispy Tofu Tacos

322 calories

¼ cup panko bread crumbs

1 tablespoon taco seasoning

½ teaspoon garlic powder

¼ teaspoon each salt and black pepper

8 ounces block-style extra-firm tofu, excess moisture removed, cut into bite-size pieces

¼ cup (about 2 large) egg whites or fat-free liquid egg substitute

¼ cup frozen sweet corn kernels

¼ cup chopped onion

¼ cup sliced zucchini

Four 6-inch corn tortillas

¼ cup salsa

2 tablespoons chopped fresh cilantro

Prep: 10 minutes

Cook: 20 minutes

You'll need:
baking sheet, nonstick spray, large sealable bag, wide bowl, paper towels

½ of recipe:
322 calories
8.5g total fat
(0.5g sat fat)
785mg sodium
39.5g carbs
4.5g fiber
5g sugars
20.5g protein

1. Preheat oven to 400 degrees. Spray a baking sheet with nonstick spray.

2. In a large sealable bag, combine panko, 2½ teaspoons taco seasoning, garlic powder, salt, and pepper.

3. Place tofu in a wide bowl. Add egg whites/substitute, and gently toss to coat.

4. Shake tofu to remove excess egg whites/substitute, and add tofu to the bag with the seasoned panko. Seal bag, and shake to coat.

5. Transfer tofu to the baking sheet. Add corn, onion, zucchini, and remaining ½ teaspoon taco seasoning. Bake until tofu is crispy and veggies are tender, about 20 minutes, flipping halfway through.

6. Place tortillas between two damp paper towels, and microwave for 15 seconds, or until warm. Fill with tofu, veggies, salsa, and cilantro.

MAKES 2 SERVINGS

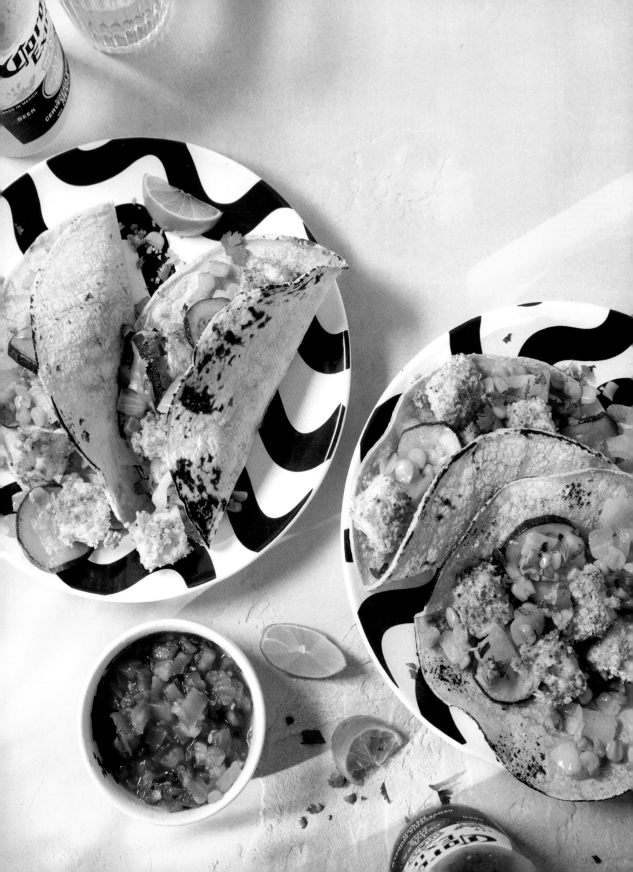

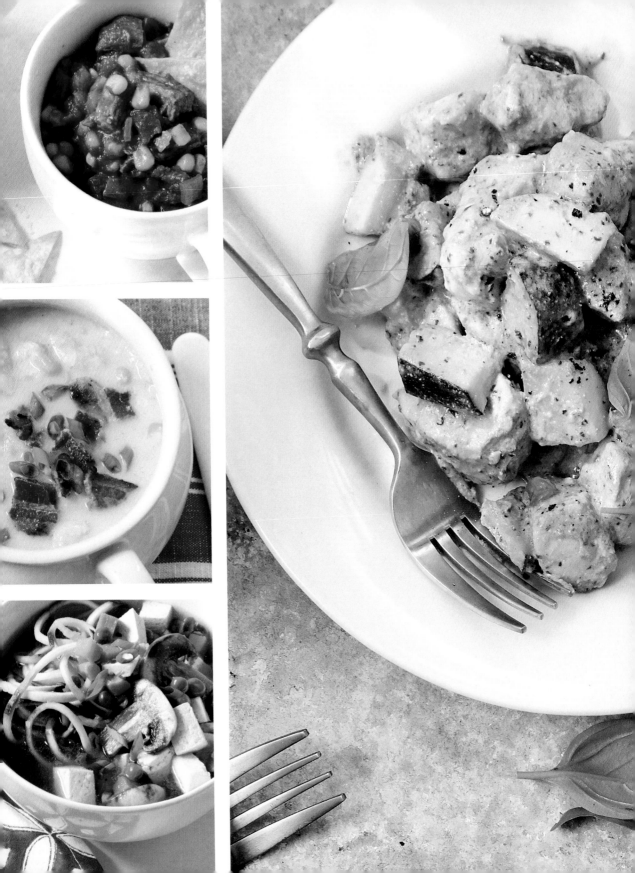

4

One-Pot Recipes

I've got more than soup and chili in my one-pot arsenal. This chapter also features Italian food, Chinese favorites, and so much more!

Creamy Chicken Soup

190 calories

3 cups frozen riced cauliflower

1½ cups fat-free milk

¾ cup chopped carrots

¾ cup chopped celery

¾ cup chopped onion

¼ cup light/reduced-fat cream cheese

1 cup reduced-sodium chicken broth

6 ounces cooked and shredded skinless chicken breast

1 teaspoon poultry seasoning

½ teaspoon dried parsley

Prep: 10 minutes

Cook: 20 minutes

You'll need:
medium microwave-safe bowl, blender or food processor, large pot, nonstick spray

¼th of recipe (about 1 cup):
190 calories
5g total fat
(2g sat fat)
340mg sodium
16.5g carbs
3.5g fiber
10g sugars
20g protein

1. In a medium microwave-safe bowl, microwave cauliflower for 3 minutes, or until thawed. Transfer to a blender or food processor. Add milk, and puree until smooth.

2. Bring a large pot sprayed with nonstick spray to medium-high heat. Add carrots, celery, and onion. Cook and stir until mostly softened, about 6 minutes. Add cream cheese, and cook and stir until melted and well mixed, about 1 minute.

3. Add cauliflower puree and remaining ingredients. Raise heat to high. Stirring occasionally, cook until veggies are tender and soup is hot and well mixed, about 6 minutes.

MAKES 4 SERVINGS

HG Tip
Grab a rotisserie chicken from the supermarket to use for recipes like this—easy to shred and so delicious!

Hungry Girl FAST & Easy

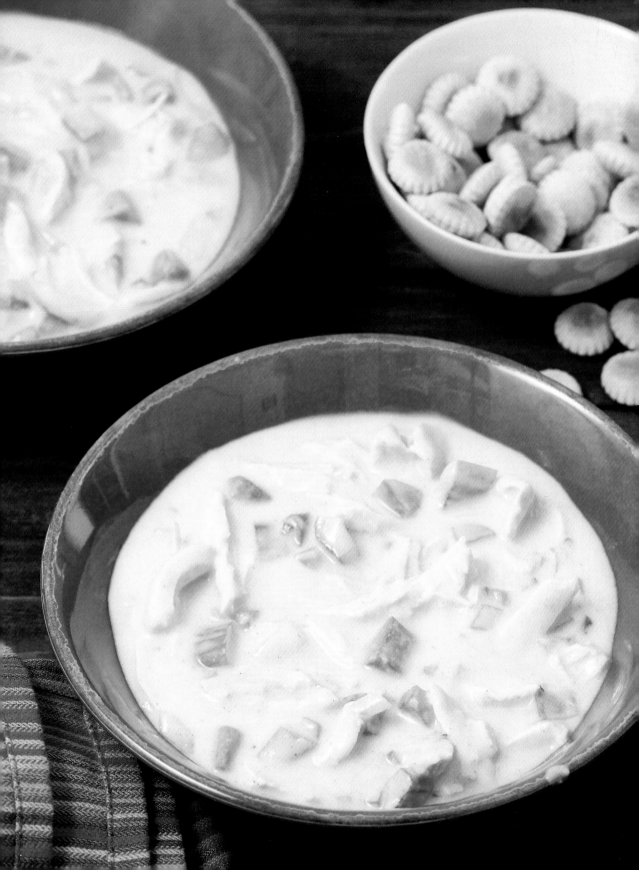

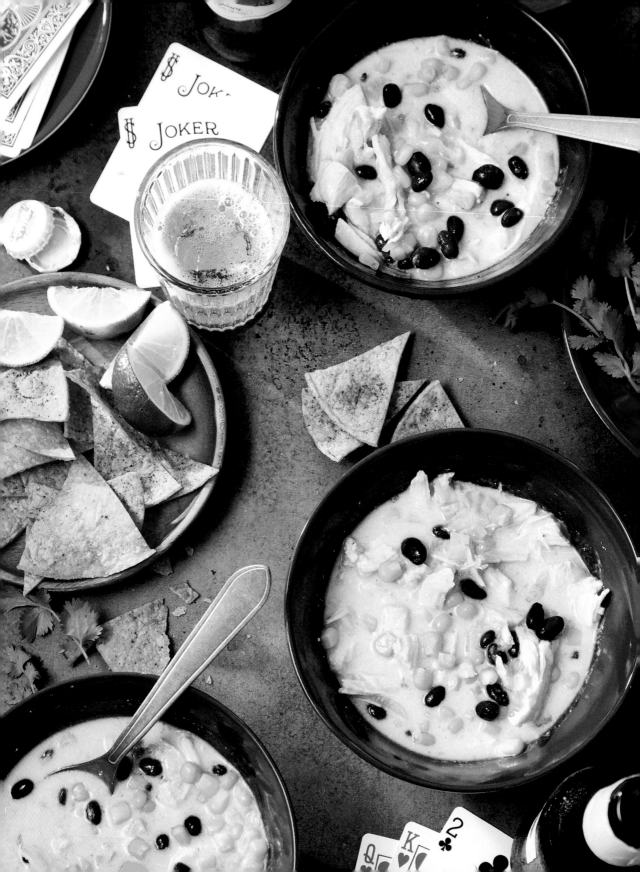

Creamy Chicken Enchilada Soup

½ cup finely chopped onion
⅔ cup green enchilada sauce
⅓ cup salsa verde
3 tablespoons light/reduced-fat cream cheese
8 ounces cooked and shredded skinless chicken breast
1½ cups reduced-sodium chicken broth
½ cup canned black beans, drained and rinsed
½ cup frozen sweet corn kernels

1. Bring a large pot sprayed with nonstick spray to medium-high heat. Add onion. Cook and stir until mostly softened, about 3 minutes.

2. Add enchilada sauce, salsa, and cream cheese. Cook and stir until melted and mixed, about 2 minutes.

3. Add remaining ingredients, and raise heat to high. Stirring occasionally, cook until onion is tender and soup is hot and well mixed, about 4 minutes.

MAKES 4 SERVINGS

30m **GF**

190 calories

Prep: 10 minutes

Cook: 10 minutes

You'll need:
large pot,
nonstick spray

**¼th of recipe
(about 1 cup):**
190 calories
5g total fat
(1.5g sat fat)
726mg sodium
15g carbs
2g fiber
4g sugars
19.5g protein

One-Pot Recipes: Poultry

Creamy Italian Chicken Stew

260 calories

I love the creaminess of this one . . . so yummy and rich!

1 cup reduced-sodium chicken broth

2½ teaspoons cornstarch

1 pound raw boneless skinless chicken breast, cut into bite-size pieces

1 cup chopped onion

1 tablespoon chopped garlic

¼ teaspoon each salt and black pepper

4 cups spinach

½ cup light/reduced-fat cream cheese

⅓ cup light/low-fat ricotta cheese

¼ cup chopped fresh basil, or more for topping

1 teaspoon Italian seasoning

1. In a medium bowl, combine broth with cornstarch. Stir to dissolve.

2. Bring a large pot sprayed with nonstick spray to medium-high heat. Add chicken, onion, garlic, salt, and pepper. Cook and stir until chicken is fully cooked and onion has mostly softened, about 6 minutes.

3. Reduce heat to medium. Add spinach, and cook and stir until wilted, about 1 minute. Add broth mixture, cream cheese, ricotta, basil, and Italian seasoning. Cook and stir until cream cheese has melted and sauce has slightly thickened, about 4 minutes.

MAKES 4 SERVINGS

Prep: 10 minutes

Cook: 15 minutes

You'll need: medium bowl, large pot, nonstick spray

¼th of recipe (about 1 cup):
260 calories
9.5g total fat
(5g sat fat)
520mg sodium
11g carbs
1.5g fiber
4g sugars
31.5g protein

One-Pot Recipes: Poultry

Hungry Girl *FAST* & Easy

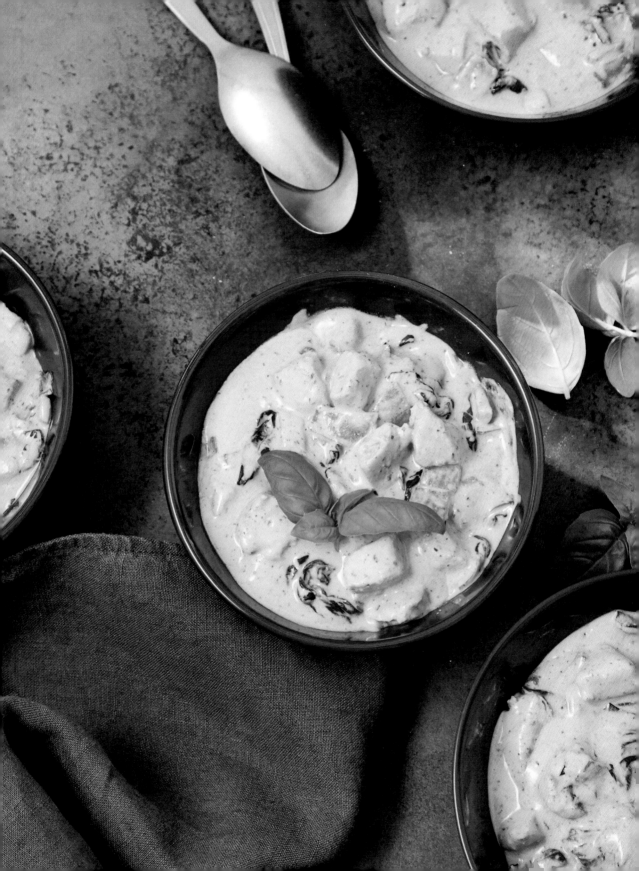

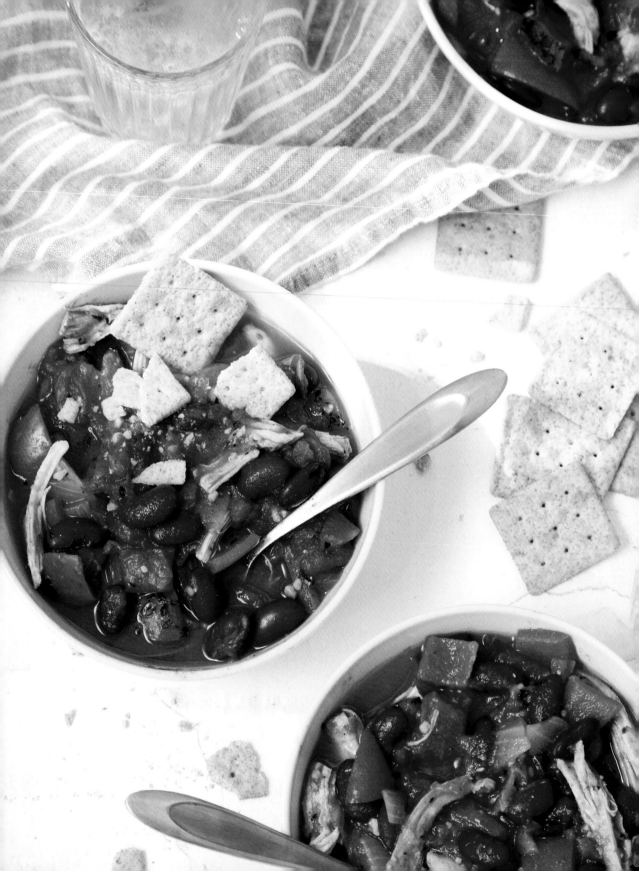

Shredded Chicken Chili

1 cup chopped red bell pepper

1 cup chopped onion

2 teaspoons chili seasoning

One 15-ounce can red kidney beans, drained and rinsed

One 14.5-ounce can fire-roasted diced tomatoes (not drained)

¾ cup canned crushed tomatoes

6 ounces cooked and shredded skinless chicken breast

2 teaspoons chopped garlic

1. Bring a large pot sprayed with nonstick spray to medium-high heat. Add pepper, onion, and 1 teaspoon chili seasoning. Cook and stir until veggies have mostly softened, about 6 minutes.

2. Add beans, fire-roasted tomatoes, crushed tomatoes, chicken, garlic, and remaining 1 teaspoon chili seasoning. Stirring occasionally, cook until veggies are tender and chili is hot and well mixed, about 2 minutes.

MAKES 4 SERVINGS

230 calories

Prep: 5 minutes

Cook: 10 minutes

You'll need:
large pot,
nonstick spray

**¼th of recipe
(about 1 cup):**
230 calories
2g total fat
(0.5g sat fat)
645mg sodium
32.5g carbs
9g fiber
10g sugars
21g protein

One-Pot Recipes: Poultry

Chunky Chicken Sausage Soup

163 calories

This satisfying soup is like a big edible hug!

9 ounces (about 3 links) fully cooked chicken sausage, sliced
    into coins
1 cup chopped onion
1 tablespoon chopped garlic
3 cups roughly chopped spinach
2 cups chopped tomatoes
2 cups low-sodium chicken broth
One 15-ounce can cannellini (white kidney) beans, drained
    and rinsed
1 teaspoon Italian seasoning

1. Bring a large pot sprayed with nonstick spray to
   medium-high heat. Add sausage, onion, and garlic.
   Cook and stir until sausage has browned and onion
   has mostly softened, about 5 minutes.

2. Add remaining ingredients, and raise heat to high.
   Stirring occasionally, cook until spinach has wilted,
   onion is tender, and soup is hot and well mixed,
   about 4 minutes.

MAKES 6 SERVINGS

30m **GF**

Prep: 10 minutes

Cook: 10 minutes

You'll need:
large pot,
nonstick spray

**⅙th of recipe
(about 1 cup):**
163 calories
4g total fat
(1g sat fat)
402mg sodium
17.5g carbs
5g fiber
3.5g sugars
13.5g protein

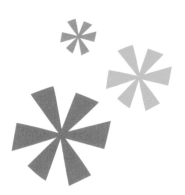

One-Pot Recipes: Poultry

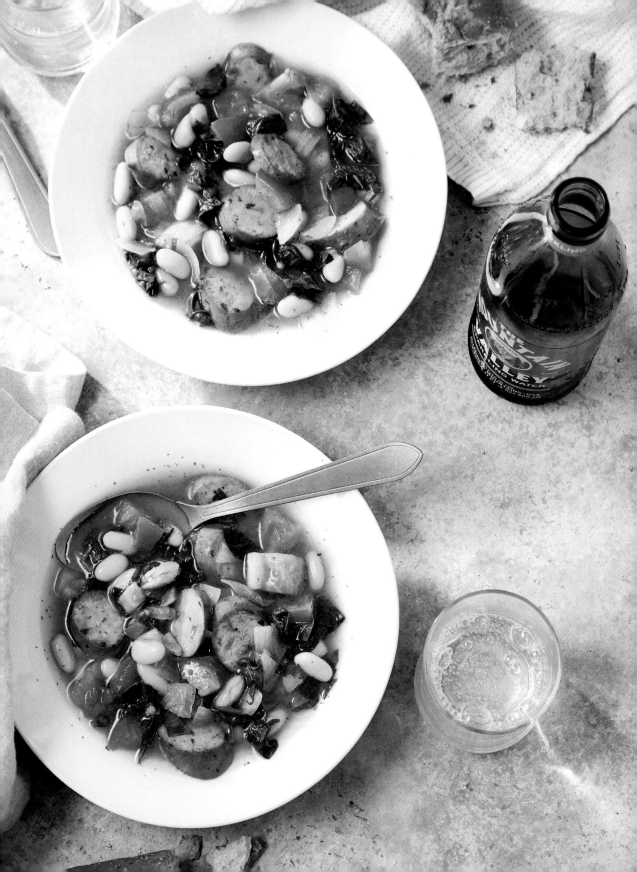

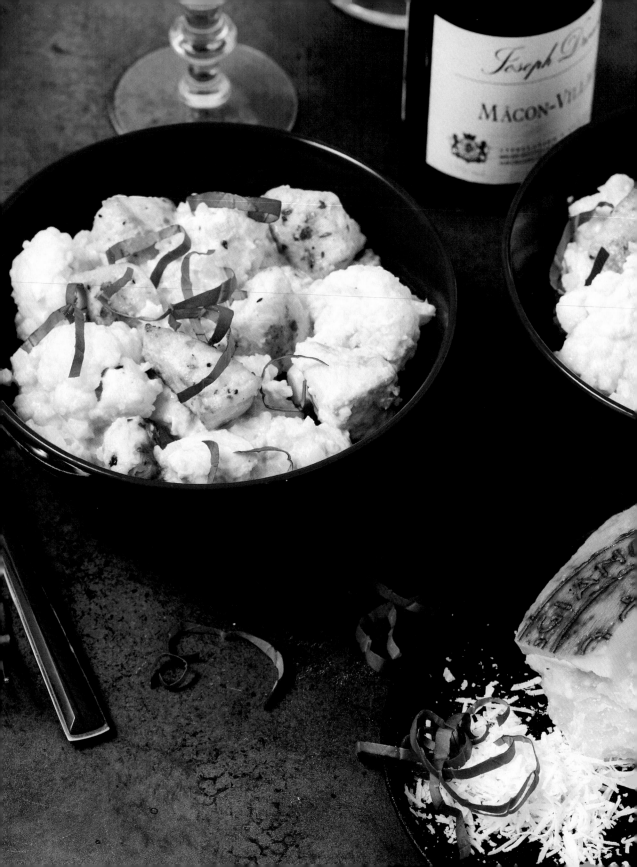

Cheesy Chicken & Cauliflower Rice

The combination of cauliflower florets and riced cauliflower is PERFECTION here!

2 cups frozen riced cauliflower

1 cup frozen cauliflower florets

1 pound raw boneless skinless chicken breast, cut into bite-size pieces

1 tablespoon chopped garlic

1 teaspoon onion powder

½ teaspoon salt

¼ teaspoon black pepper

½ cup light/reduced-fat cream cheese

2 tablespoons whipped butter

2 tablespoons grated Parmesan cheese

Optional topping: fresh basil

1. Bring a large pot sprayed with nonstick spray to medium-high heat. Add riced cauliflower and cauliflower florets. Cover and cook for 4 minutes, or until thawed.

2. Add chicken, garlic, onion powder, salt, and pepper. Cook and stir for about 6 minutes, until chicken is fully cooked.

3. Reduce heat to medium. Add cream cheese, butter, and Parm. Cook and stir until melted and well mixed, about 2 minutes.

MAKES 4 SERVINGS

282 calories

Prep: 5 minutes

Cook: 15 minutes

You'll need:
large pot with lid, nonstick spray

¼th of recipe (about 1 cup):
282 calories
13.5g total fat
(7g sat fat)
602mg sodium
8g carbs
2g fiber
3.5g sugars
31.5g protein

Lemon & Herb Chicken & Veggies

248 calories

Fresh, light, and filling . . . What more could you want from a one-pot meal?

Prep: 10 minutes

Cook: 15 minutes

You'll need:
large pot,
nonstick spray

**¼th of recipe
(about 1 cup):**
248 calories
9.5g total fat
(4.5g sat fat)
398mg sodium
12g carbs
3g fiber
5g sugars
28g protein

1 pound raw boneless skinless chicken breast, cut into
    bite-size pieces
1½ cups chopped sweet onion
½ teaspoon dried oregano
½ teaspoon each salt and black pepper
¼ teaspoon dried thyme
2 cups asparagus cut into 1-inch pieces
1 cup cherry tomatoes, halved
¼ cup whipped butter
3 tablespoons lemon juice
1 tablespoon chopped garlic
1 teaspoon lemon zest

1. Bring a large pot sprayed with nonstick spray
   to medium-high heat. Add chicken, onion, and
   seasonings. Cook and stir until chicken is lightly
   browned, about 4 minutes.

2. Add remaining ingredients. Cook and stir until
   chicken is fully cooked and veggies are tender,
   about 6 minutes.

MAKES 4 SERVINGS

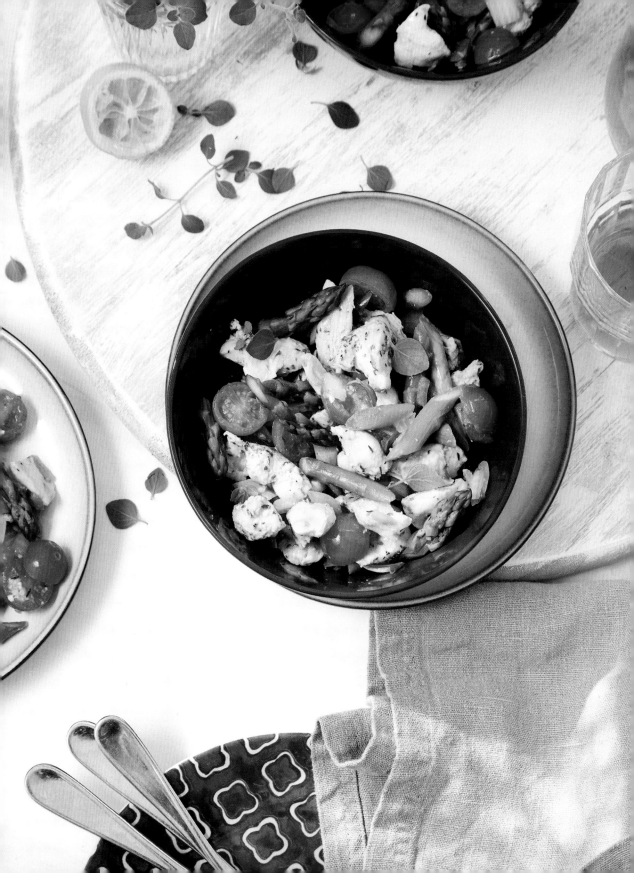

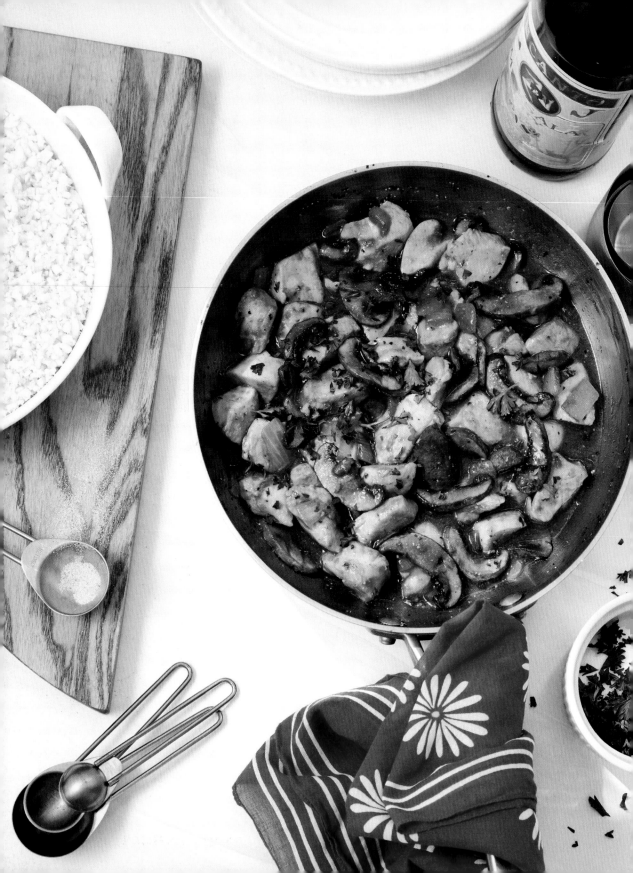

I love this one! It's perfect over cauliflower rice . . .

230 calories

2 tablespoons whipped butter
½ cup marsala wine
1 tablespoon cornstarch
1 pound raw boneless skinless chicken breast, cut into bite-size pieces
2 cups sliced brown mushrooms
½ cup chopped onion
¼ teaspoon garlic powder
½ teaspoon salt
¼ teaspoon black pepper
Optional topping: parsley

1. In a medium microwave-safe bowl, microwave butter for 20 seconds, or until melted. Add wine and cornstarch, and stir to dissolve. (Whisk, if needed.)

2. Bring a large pot sprayed with nonstick spray to medium-high heat. Add chicken, mushrooms, onion, garlic powder, salt, and pepper. Cook and stir until chicken is lightly browned, about 5 minutes.

3. Reduce heat to medium. Add wine mixture, and cook and stir until chicken is fully cooked, veggies are tender, and sauce has thickened, about 5 minutes.

MAKES 4 SERVINGS

Prep: 5 minutes

Cook: 15 minutes

You'll need: medium microwave-safe bowl, large pot, nonstick spray

¼th of recipe (about 1 cup):
230 calories
6.5g total fat
(2.5g sat fat)
554mg sodium
10.5g carbs
0.5g fiber
5g sugars
26.5g protein

One-Pot Recipes: Poultry

Creamy Salsa Chicken

232 calories

Classic flavors perfected, and just seven simple ingredients!

1 pound raw boneless skinless chicken breast, cut into bite-size pieces
1 tablespoon taco seasoning
2 cups chopped red bell peppers
1 cup chopped onion
1 cup salsa
½ cup chopped fresh cilantro, or more for topping
¼ cup light/reduced-fat cream cheese

1. Bring a large pot sprayed with nonstick spray to medium-high heat. Add chicken and taco seasoning. Cook and stir until lightly browned, about 4 minutes.

2. Add peppers and onion. Cook and stir until chicken is fully cooked and veggies have softened, about 6 minutes.

3. Reduce heat to medium. Add salsa, cilantro, and cream cheese. Cook and stir until melted and well mixed, about 3 minutes.

MAKES 4 SERVINGS

  30m GF

Prep: 10 minutes

Cook: 15 minutes

You'll need:
large pot,
nonstick spray

**¼th of recipe
(about 1 cup):**
232 calories
6g total fat
(2.5g sat fat)
600mg sodium
15g carbs
2.5g fiber
8.5g sugars
28g protein

One-Pot Recipes: Poultry

Hungry Girl FAST & Easy

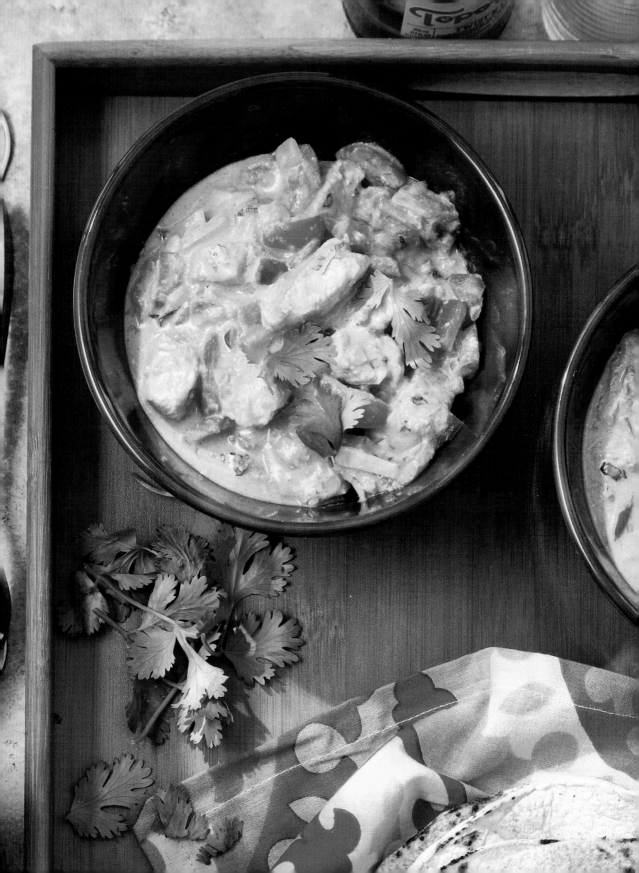

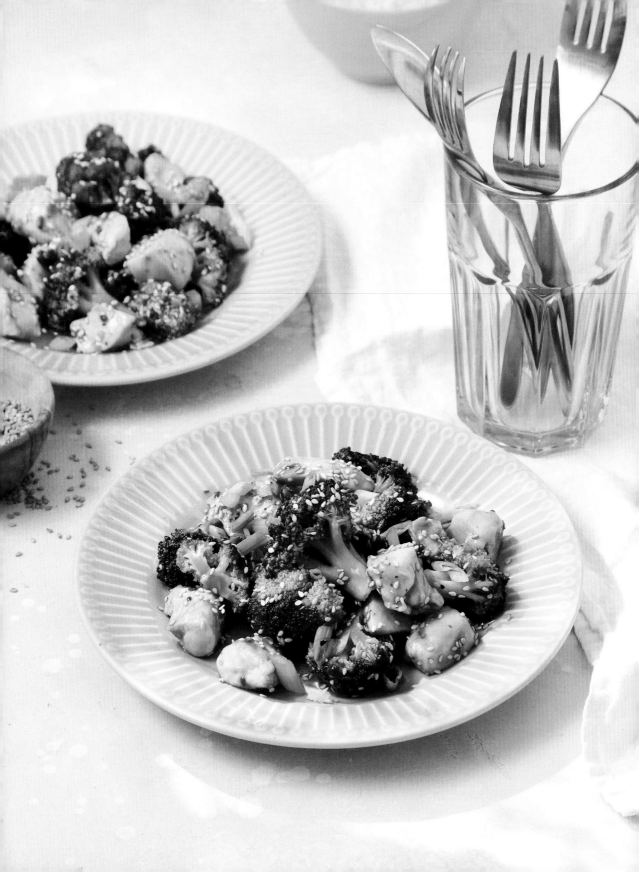

Sesame Chicken

Chinese food in 20 minutes? This one's faster than delivery, and a lot healthier too . . .

1 tablespoon cornstarch
1 tablespoon seasoned rice vinegar
1 tablespoon sesame oil
⅓ cup thick teriyaki sauce or marinade
5 cups frozen broccoli florets
1 pound raw boneless skinless chicken breast, cut into bite-size pieces
⅛ teaspoon each salt and black pepper
2 teaspoons chopped garlic
⅓ cup chopped scallions
1 tablespoon sesame seeds

1. In a small bowl, combine cornstarch, vinegar, and oil. Stir to dissolve. Add teriyaki, and mix well.

2. Bring a large pot sprayed with nonstick spray to medium-high heat. Add broccoli. Cover and cook for 5 minutes, or until mostly thawed.

3. Add chicken, salt, and pepper. Cook and stir until broccoli is hot and chicken is fully cooked, about 6 minutes.

4. Reduce heat to medium. Add teriyaki mixture and garlic. Cook and stir until slightly thickened, about 2 minutes.

5. Serve topped with scallions and sesame seeds.

MAKES 4 SERVINGS

30m

265 calories

Prep: 5 minutes

Cook: 15 minutes

You'll need: small bowl, large pot with lid, nonstick spray

¼th of recipe (about 1 cup):
265 calories
8g total fat
(1g sat fat)
792mg sodium
18g carbs
3.5g fiber
8g sugars
29g protein

One-Pot Recipes: Poultry

Garlic Parm Chicken

279 calories

This dish is to DIE for! I've been enjoying it over zucchini noodles . . .

1 pound raw boneless skinless chicken breast, cut into bite-size pieces
1 cup chopped onion
½ teaspoon onion powder
¼ teaspoon each salt and black pepper
2 cups chopped mushrooms
1 tablespoon chopped garlic
5 cups roughly chopped spinach
½ cup light/reduced-fat cream cheese
¼ cup grated Parmesan cheese

1. Bring a large pot sprayed with nonstick spray to medium-high heat. Add chicken, onion, onion powder, salt, and pepper. Cook and stir until lightly browned, about 4 minutes.

2. Add mushrooms and garlic. Cook and stir until chicken is fully cooked and veggies have mostly softened, about 3 minutes.

3. Add spinach, and cook and stir until wilted, about 1 minute.

4. Reduce heat to medium-low. Add cream cheese and Parm. Cook and stir until melted and well mixed, about 2 minutes.

MAKES 4 SERVINGS

Prep: 10 minutes

Cook: 10 minutes

You'll need:
large pot,
nonstick spray

¼th of recipe (about 1 cup):
279 calories
11.5g total fat
(6g sat fat)
511mg sodium
9.5g carbs
2g fiber
4g sugars
34g protein

One-Pot Recipes: Poultry

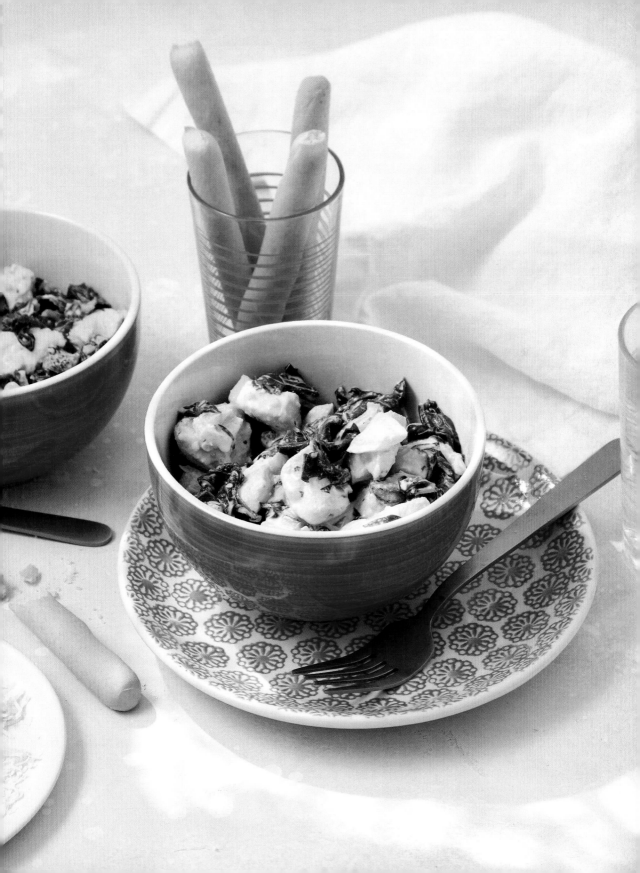

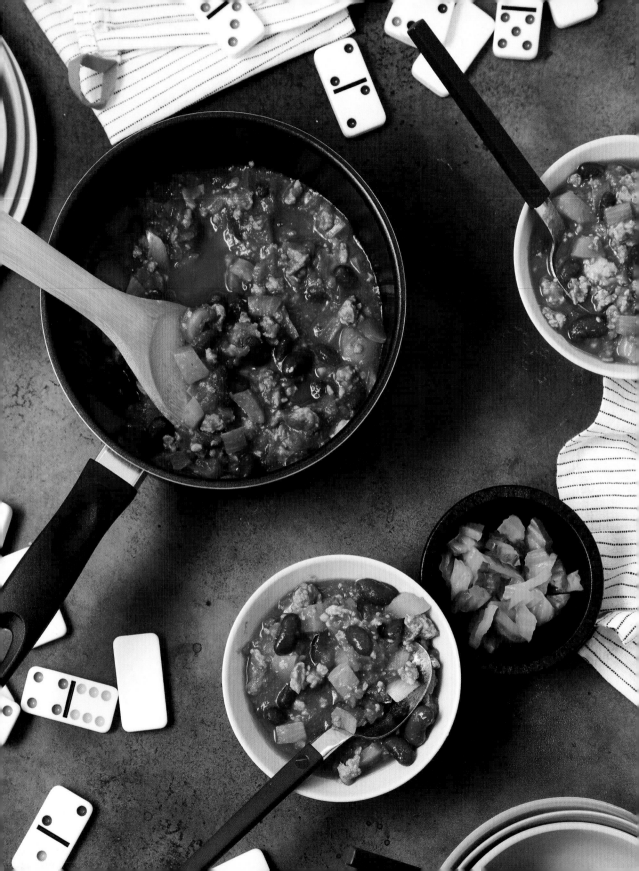

This is one of my favorite Hungry Girl chili recipes to date! Meaning it's a favorite so far. I don't want to take it to the movies . . .

12 ounces raw extra-lean ground turkey (at least 98% lean)
1 cup chopped bell pepper
1 cup chopped onion
2 teaspoons chili seasoning
One 15-ounce can red kidney beans, drained and rinsed
One 14.5-ounce can diced tomatoes (not drained)
1 cup canned crushed tomatoes
3 tablespoons ketchup
1 tablespoon chopped garlic
2 teaspoons yellow mustard
Optional topping: chopped pickles

1. Bring a large pot sprayed with nonstick spray to medium-high heat. Add turkey, pepper, onion, and 1 teaspoon chili seasoning. Cook and crumble until turkey is fully cooked and veggies have mostly softened, about 7 minutes.

2. Add remaining ingredients, including remaining 1 teaspoon chili seasoning. Stirring occasionally, cook until veggies are tender and chili is hot and well mixed, about 2 minutes.

MAKES 5 SERVINGS

30m **GF**

215 calories

Prep: 10 minutes

Cook: 10 minutes

You'll need:
large pot,
nonstick spray

**⅕th of recipe
(about 1 cup):**
215 calories
1g total fat
(0g sat fat)
631mg sodium
29.5g carbs
7.5g fiber
10.5g sugars
23g protein

One-Pot Recipes: Poultry

Chicken Cacciatore Soup

165 calories

The beloved Italian entrée, reimagined as a soup. So great!

12 ounces raw boneless skinless chicken breast, cut into bite-size pieces
1 cup chopped bell pepper
1 cup chopped onion
½ teaspoon garlic powder
½ teaspoon Italian seasoning
2 cups chopped mushrooms
3½ cups reduced-sodium creamy tomato soup with 140 calories or less per cup
1 tablespoon grated Parmesan cheese
Optional topping: chopped fresh basil

1. Bring a large pot sprayed with nonstick spray to medium-high heat. Add chicken, pepper, onion, garlic powder, and Italian seasoning. Cook and stir until lightly browned, about 4 minutes.

2. Add mushrooms. Cook and stir until chicken is fully cooked and veggies have mostly softened, about 5 minutes.

3. Add soup and Parm. Stirring occasionally, cook until veggies are tender and soup is hot and well mixed, about 2 minutes.

MAKES 6 SERVINGS

Prep: 10 minutes

Cook: 15 minutes

You'll need: large pot, nonstick spray

⅙th of recipe (about 1 cup):
165 calories
3.5g total fat
(1.5g sat fat)
269mg sodium
17g carbs
2g fiber
10g sugars
16.5g protein

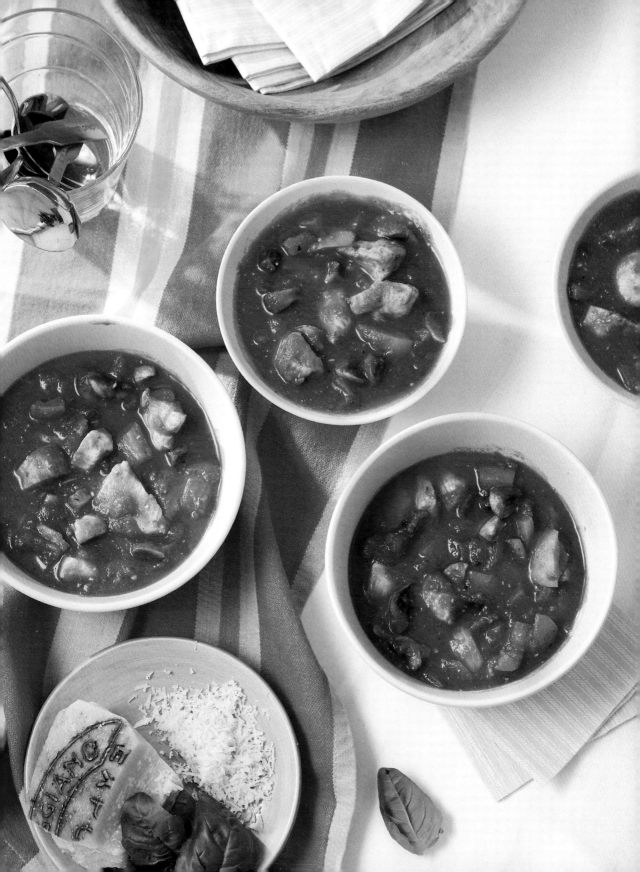

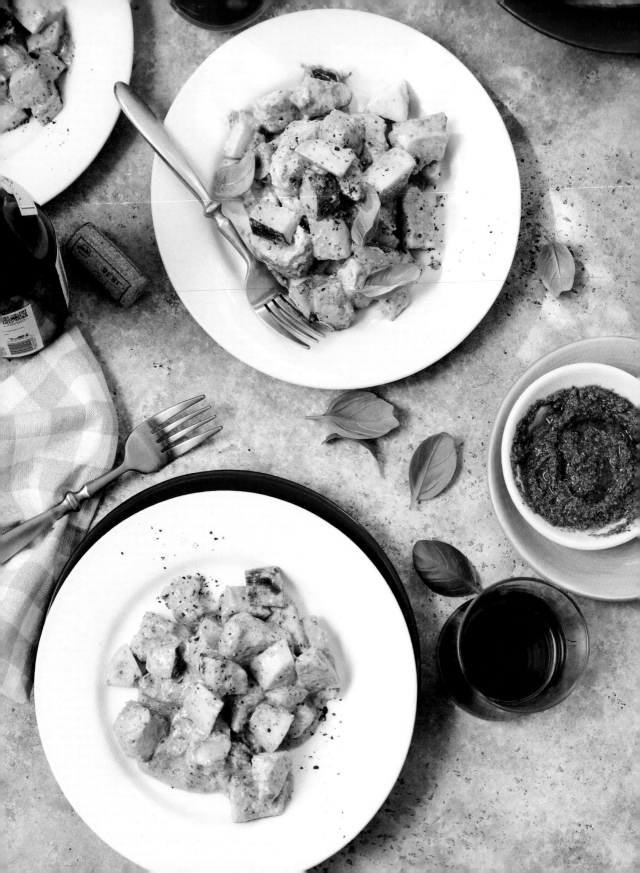

Creamy Pesto Chicken

1 pound raw boneless skinless chicken breast, cut into
   bite-size pieces

1 cup chopped onion

⅛ teaspoon each salt and black pepper

1 cup roughly chopped yellow squash

1 cup roughly chopped zucchini

½ cup pesto sauce

½ cup light/low-fat ricotta cheese

¼ cup light/reduced-fat cream cheese, room temperature

Optional topping: fresh basil

1. Bring a large pot sprayed with nonstick spray to
   medium-high heat. Add chicken, onion, salt, and
   pepper. Cook and stir until lightly browned, about
   4 minutes.

2. Add squash and zucchini. Cook and stir until chicken
   is fully cooked and veggies have softened, about
   5 minutes.

3. Reduce heat to medium-low. Add pesto, ricotta, and
   cream cheese. Cook and stir until melted and well
   mixed, about 2 minutes.

MAKES 4 SERVINGS

 GF

352 calories

Prep: 10 minutes

Cook: 15 minutes

You'll need:
large pot,
nonstick spray

**¼th of recipe
(about 1 cup):**
352 calories
19.5g total fat
(5.5g sat fat)
47mg sodium
11g carbs
1.5g fiber
6g sugars
32.5g protein

HG Tip
Use that leftover pesto to make the Pesto Zucchini-Noodle Salad on page 71!

One-Pot Recipes: Poultry

Orange Chicken

264 calories

5 cups frozen broccoli florets
2 tablespoons reduced-sodium/lite soy sauce
1 tablespoon cornstarch
1 pound raw boneless skinless chicken breast, cut into
    bite-size pieces
1 teaspoon onion powder
¼ teaspoon each salt and black pepper
⅓ cup orange marmalade
2 teaspoons chopped garlic
¼ cup chopped scallions

30m

Prep: 10 minutes

Cook: 15 minutes

You'll need:
large pot with lid,
nonstick spray,
small bowl

**¼th of recipe
(about 1 cup):**
264 calories
3g total fat
(0.5g sat fat)
495mg sodium
27g carbs
3g fiber
19g sugars
29g protein

1. Bring a large pot sprayed with nonstick spray to
   medium-high heat. Add broccoli. Cover and cook for
   5 minutes, or until mostly thawed.

2. Meanwhile, in a small bowl, combine soy sauce with
   cornstarch. Stir to dissolve.

3. Add chicken, onion powder, salt, and pepper to the
   pot. Cook and stir until broccoli is hot and chicken is
   fully cooked, about 7 minutes.

4. Reduce heat to medium. Add marmalade, soy sauce
   mixture, and garlic. Cook and stir until sauce has
   thickened, about 2 minutes.

5. Serve topped with scallions.

MAKES 4 SERVINGS

One-Pot Recipes: Poultry

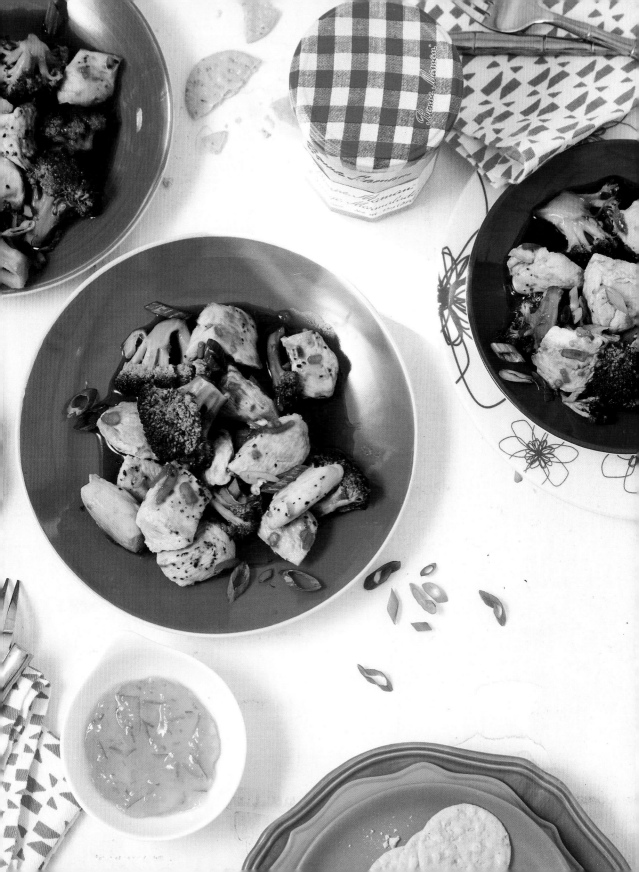

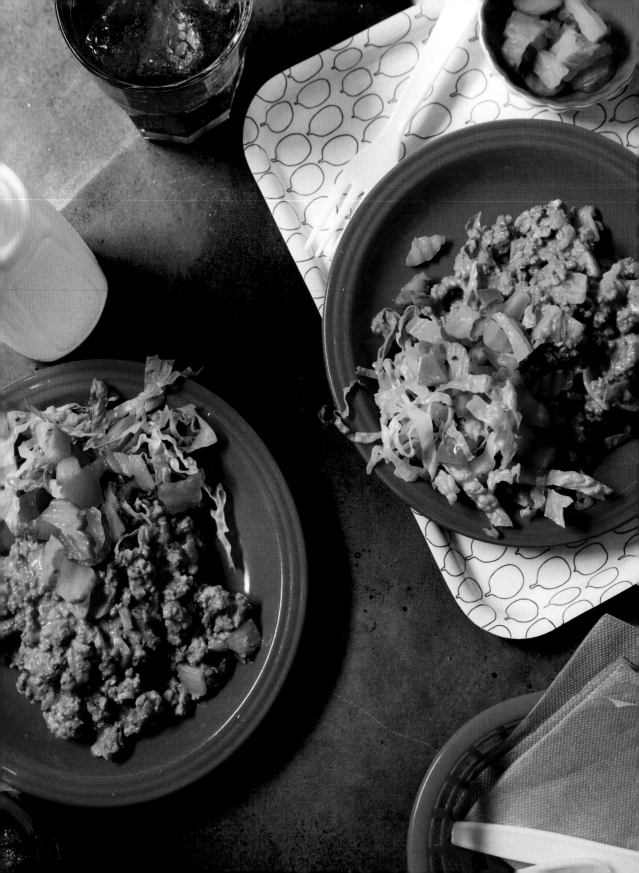

Cheeseburger Heaven

This recipe is aptly named ... It tastes like heaven in a bowl! Serve it over shredded lettuce, and you've got one blissfully delicious meal.

1 pound raw extra-lean ground beef (at least 96% lean)
1 cup chopped onion
1 teaspoon garlic powder
¼ teaspoon each salt and black pepper
⅓ cup shredded reduced-fat cheddar cheese
⅓ cup light/reduced-fat cream cheese
3 tablespoons ketchup
1 tablespoon yellow mustard
Optional toppings: chopped tomatoes, chopped pickles

1. Bring a large pot sprayed with nonstick spray to medium-high heat. Add beef, onion, garlic powder, salt, and pepper. Cook and crumble until beef is fully cooked and onion has mostly softened, about 5 minutes.

2. Reduce heat to medium. Add remaining ingredients. Cook and stir until melted and well mixed, about 2 minutes.

MAKES 4 SERVINGS

Prep: 5 minutes

Cook: 10 minutes

251 calories

You'll need:
large pot, nonstick spray

¼th of recipe (about ¾ cup):
251 calories
10.5g total fat
(5.5g sat fat)
543mg sodium
10g carbs
1g fiber
45.5g sugars
2g protein

One-Pot Recipes: Beef & Pork

Steak Tamale Stew

247 calories

The flavor of this stew reminds me so much of the inside of a beef tamale! It can be yours in a fast 15 minutes . . .

Prep: 5 minutes

Cook: 10 minutes

You'll need:
large pot,
nonstick spray

¼th of recipe (about 1¼ cups):
247 calories
7.5g total fat
(3g sat fat)
577mg sodium
21.5g carbs
3.5g fiber
9.5g sugars
23g protein

12 ounces raw lean flank steak, cut into bite-size pieces
1 cup chopped onion
1 tablespoon chili powder
2 teaspoons ground cumin
Dash each salt and black pepper
One 14.5-ounce can diced tomatoes with green chiles (not drained)
1 cup reduced-sodium creamy tomato soup with 140 calories or less per cup
1 cup frozen sweet corn kernels

1. Bring a large pot sprayed with nonstick spray to medium-high heat. Add steak, onion, chili powder, cumin, salt, and pepper. Cook and stir until steak is fully cooked and onion has mostly softened, about 3 minutes.

2. Add tomatoes with chiles, soup, and corn. Raise heat to high. Stirring occasionally, cook until onion is tender and stew is hot and well mixed, about 2 minutes.

MAKES 4 SERVINGS

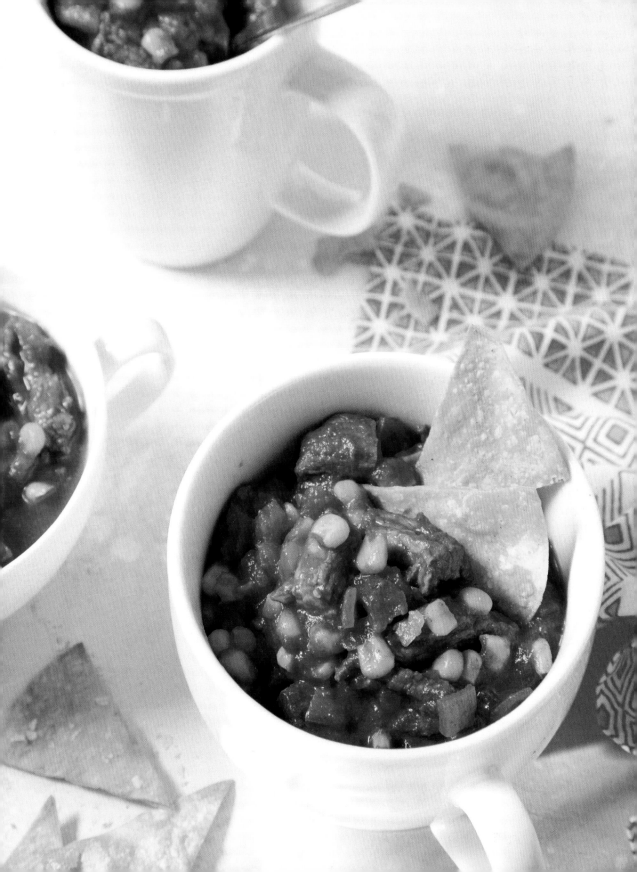

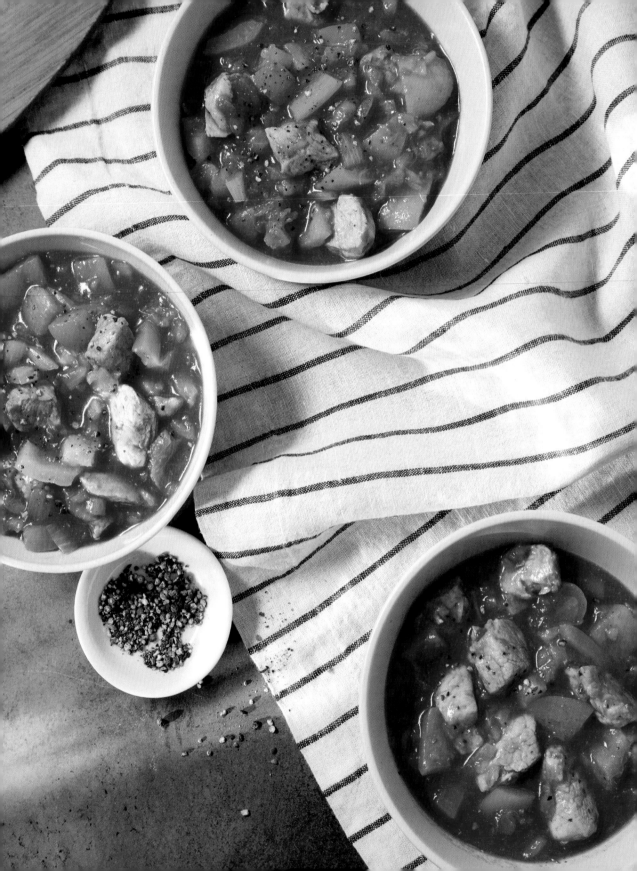

Hawaiian BBQ Pork

Pork tenderloin is underrated and underused. I love it in this recipe with the pineapple and BBQ sauce!

Prep: 5 minutes

Cook: 15 minutes

You'll need:
large pot,
nonstick spray

**¼th of recipe
(about 1½ cups):**
328 calories
4g total fat
(1g sat fat)
738mg sodium
48g carbs
4.5g fiber
34.5g sugars
26.5g protein

328 calories

1 pound raw lean boneless pork tenderloin, cut into
    bite-size pieces
⅛ teaspoon each salt and black pepper
1½ cups chopped bell peppers
1½ cups chopped onion
One 20-ounce can crushed pineapple packed in juice, drained
1 cup canned crushed tomatoes
⅔ cup BBQ sauce with 45 calories or less per 2-tablespoon
    serving
2 teaspoons garlic powder

1. Bring a large pot sprayed with nonstick spray to
   medium-high heat. Add pork, salt, and black pepper.
   Cook and stir until lightly browned, about 5 minutes.

2. Add bell peppers and onion. Cook and stir until pork
   is fully cooked and veggies have softened, about
   6 minutes.

3. Add remaining ingredients. Cook and stir until hot and
   well mixed, about 2 minutes.

MAKES 4 SERVINGS

Mexican Steak Stew

194 calories

1½ cups chopped carrots

1 cup chopped onion

12 ounces raw lean flank steak, cut in bite-size pieces

1 tablespoon chopped garlic

¼ teaspoon each salt and black pepper

One 14.5-ounce can diced tomatoes with green chiles (not drained)

1 cup reduced-sodium beef broth

½ cup chopped fresh cilantro, or more for topping

1½ teaspoons chili powder

1 teaspoon ground cumin

 30m **GF**

Prep: 10 minutes

Cook: 15 minutes

You'll need:
large pot with lid,
nonstick spray

**¼th of recipe
(about 1⅓ cups):**
194 calories
6g total fat
(2g sat fat)
678mg sodium
14g carbs
3.5g fiber
6.5g sugars
21.5g protein

1. Bring a large pot sprayed with nonstick spray to medium-high heat. Add carrots, onion, and ⅓ cup water. Cover and cook for 5 minutes, until mostly softened.

2. Add steak, garlic, salt, and pepper. Cook and stir until seared on all sides, about 3 minutes.

3. Add remaining ingredients, and raise heat to high. Stirring occasionally, cook until veggies are tender and steak is fully cooked, about 2 minutes.

MAKES 4 SERVINGS

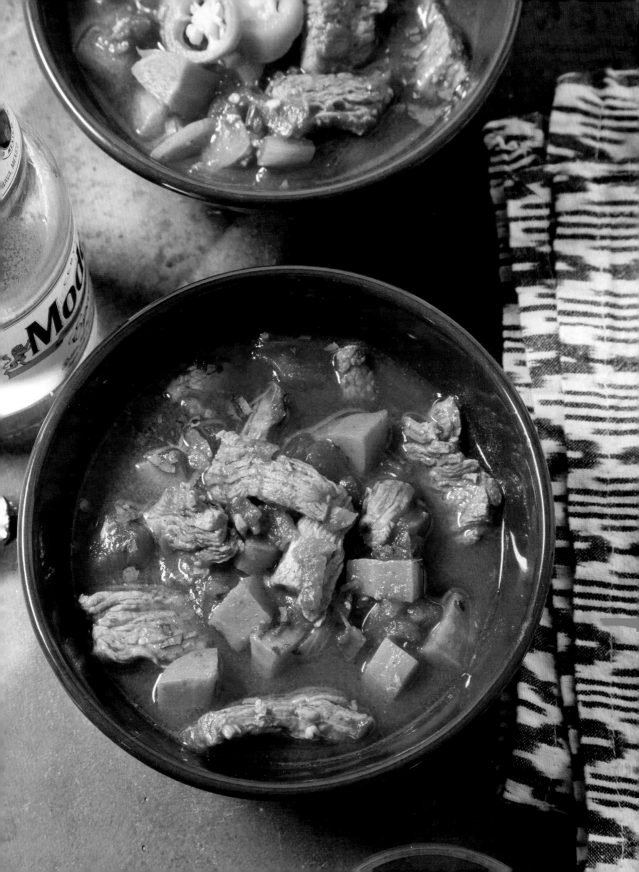

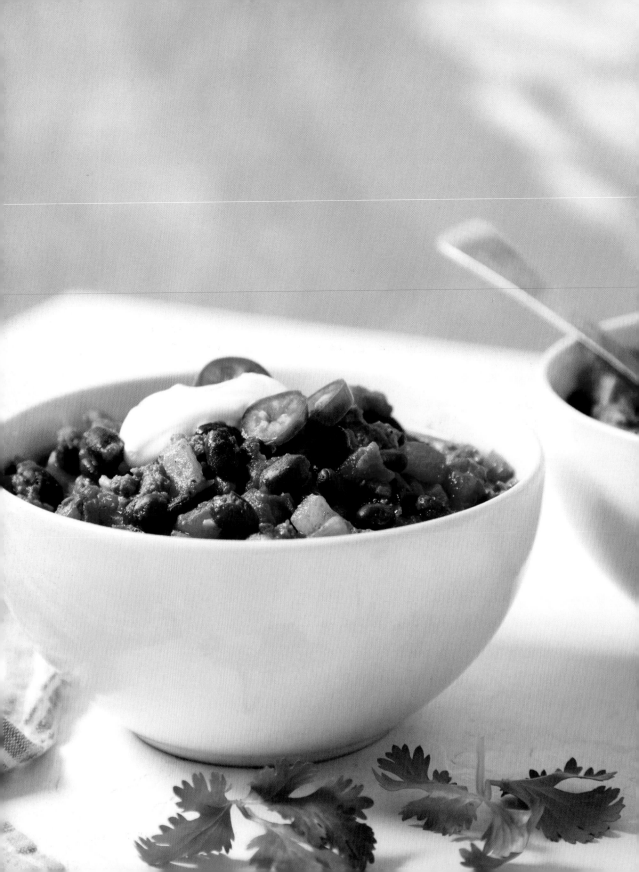

Black Bean & Beef Chili

12 ounces raw extra-lean ground beef (at least 96% lean)
1 cup chopped red bell pepper
1 cup chopped red onion
1 tablespoon chili powder
One 15-ounce can black beans, drained and rinsed
One 14.5-ounce can fire-roasted diced tomatoes (not drained)
1 cup canned crushed tomatoes
1 tablespoon chopped garlic
1 teaspoon ground cumin
Optional toppings: light sour cream, jalapeño slices

1. Bring a large pot sprayed with nonstick spray to medium-high heat. Add beef, pepper, onion, and 1 teaspoon chili powder. Cook and crumble until beef is fully cooked and veggies have mostly softened, about 6 minutes.

2. Add remaining ingredients, including the remaining 2 teaspoons chili powder. Raise heat to high. Stirring occasionally, cook until veggies are tender and chili is hot and well mixed, about 4 minutes.

MAKES 6 SERVINGS

180 calories

Prep: 5 minutes

Cook: 15 minutes

You'll need:
large pot,
nonstick spray

⅙th recipe
(about 1 cup):
180 calories
3g total fat
(1g sat fat)
417mg sodium
21g carbs
6g fiber
6g sugars
17g protein

One-Pot Recipes: Beef & Pork

World's Easiest Cioppino

243 calories

My husband LOVES cioppino, but he can be pretty picky. Luckily, this simple seafood stew has earned his seal of approval!

½ cup chopped bell pepper
½ cup chopped onion
6 ounces raw cod, cut into chunks
6 ounces (about 4) raw small scallops
6 ounces (about 8) raw large shrimp, peeled, tails removed, deveined
2 teaspoons chopped garlic
¼ teaspoon dried oregano
3½ cups reduced-sodium creamy tomato soup with 140 calories or less per cup
One 6.5-ounce can chopped clams in juice (not drained)
Optional topping: chopped fresh basil

1. Bring a large pot sprayed with nonstick spray to medium-high heat. Add pepper, onion, and ¼ cup water. Cover and cook for 4 minutes, or until mostly softened.

2. Add cod, scallops, shrimp, garlic, and oregano. Cook and stir until fully cooked, about 4 minutes.

3. Add soup and clams, and raise heat to high. Stirring occasionally, cook until hot and well mixed, about 3 minutes.

MAKES 4 SERVINGS

Prep: 10 minutes

Cook: 15 minutes

You'll need:
large pot with lid, nonstick spray

¼th of recipe (about 1½ cups):
243 calories
3g total fat
(1g sat fat)
869mg sodium
24.5g carbs
2g fiber
13g sugars
28g protein

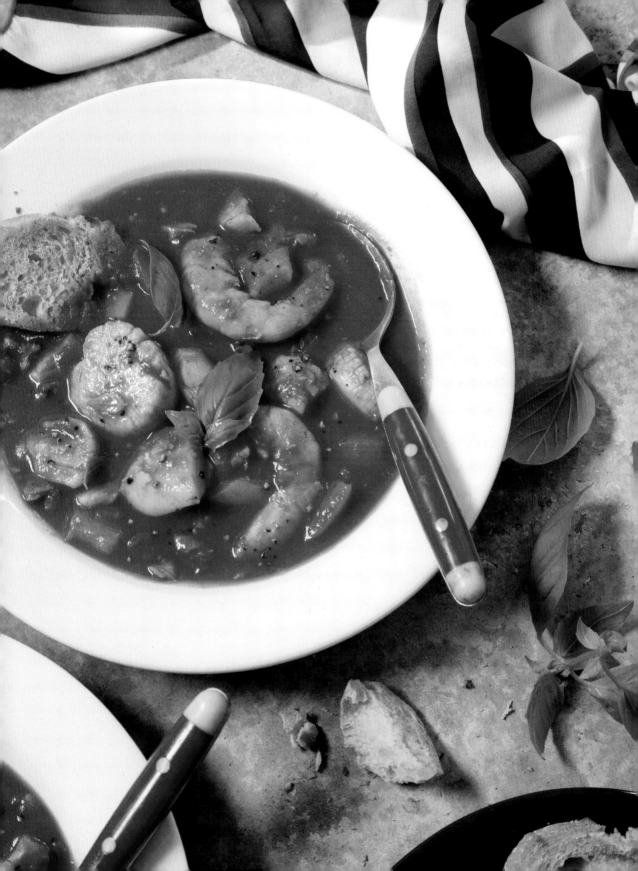

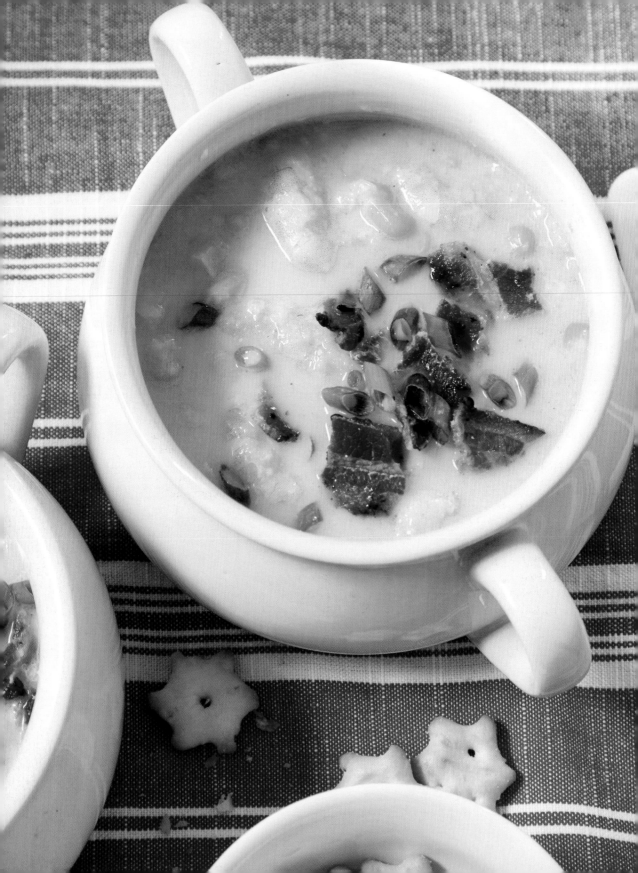

Shrimp & Bacon Corn Chowder

Bacon & shrimp . . . an unexpected (and delicious) love story!

3 slices center-cut bacon or turkey bacon

2½ cups frozen sweet corn kernels

2 cups frozen riced cauliflower

1½ cups fat-free milk

1 cup chopped sweet onion

1 cup reduced-sodium chicken broth

6 ounces (about 12 large) ready-to-eat shrimp, chopped

2 teaspoons chopped garlic

1 teaspoon onion powder

¼ teaspoon each salt and black pepper

¼ cup chopped scallions

1. Cook bacon until crispy, either in a skillet over medium heat or on a microwave-safe plate in the microwave. Roughly chop, and set aside for topping.

2. Place 1½ cups corn in a medium-large microwave-safe bowl. Add cauliflower, cover, and microwave for 4 minutes, or until thawed. Transfer to a blender or food processor. Add milk, and puree until smooth.

3. Bring a large pot sprayed with nonstick spray to medium-high heat. Add onion, and cook and stir until mostly softened, about 4 minutes.

4. Add cauliflower-corn puree, broth, shrimp, garlic, seasonings, and remaining 1 cup corn. Raise heat to high. Stirring occasionally, cook until onion is tender and soup is hot and well mixed, about 5 minutes.

5. Serve topped with bacon and scallions.

MAKES 5 SERVINGS

Prep: 10 minutes

Cook: 20 minutes

You'll need:
skillet or microwave-safe plate, medium-large microwave-safe bowl, blender or food processor, large pot, nonstick spray

⅕th of recipe (about 1 cup):
186 calories
3g total fat
(0.5g sat fat)
458mg sodium
25.5g carbs
3g fiber
10g sugars
16g protein

186 calories

One-Pot Recipes: Seafood

Cajun Salmon Chowder

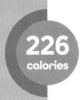

226 calories

2 cups frozen diced potatoes
1 cup chopped bell pepper
1 cup chopped onion
½ cup chopped celery
10 ounces raw skinless salmon, cut into bite-size pieces
1 tablespoon chopped garlic
1 cup low-sodium chicken broth
1 cup canned fire-roasted diced tomatoes (not drained)
½ cup light/reduced-fat cream cheese
2 teaspoons Cajun seasoning

1. Bring a large pot sprayed with nonstick spray to medium-high heat. Add potatoes, pepper, onion, celery, and ½ cup water. Cover and cook for 6 minutes, or until mostly softened.

2. Add salmon and garlic. Cook and stir until salmon is fully cooked, about 5 minutes.

3. Add remaining ingredients. Raise heat to high. Stirring occasionally, cook until veggies are tender and chowder is hot and well mixed, about 3 minutes.

MAKES 5 SERVINGS

Prep: 10 minutes

Cook: 15 minutes

You'll need:
large pot with lid, nonstick spray

⅕th of recipe (about 1 cup):
226 calories
9.5g total fat
(4g sat fat)
404mg sodium
19.5g carbs
3g fiber
5g sugars
16g protein

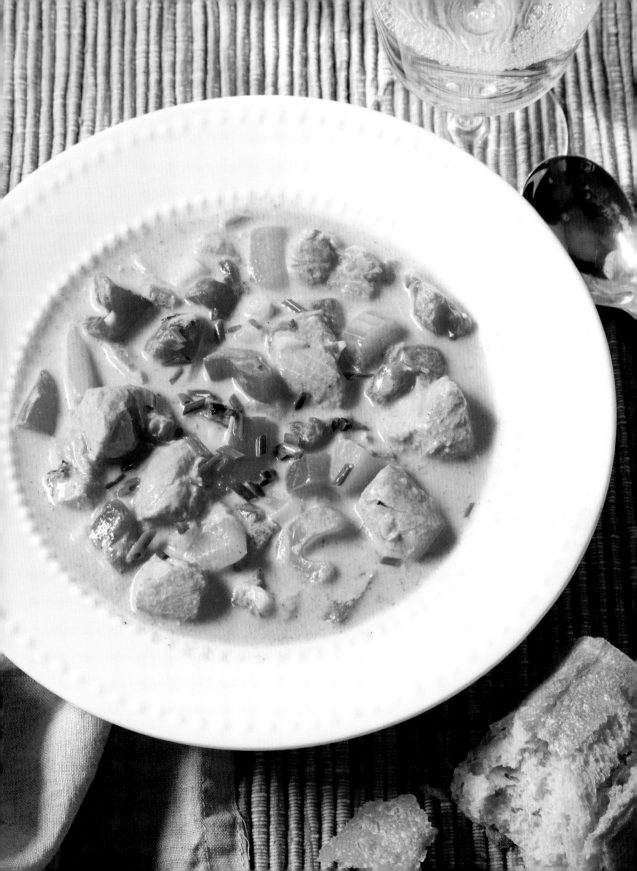

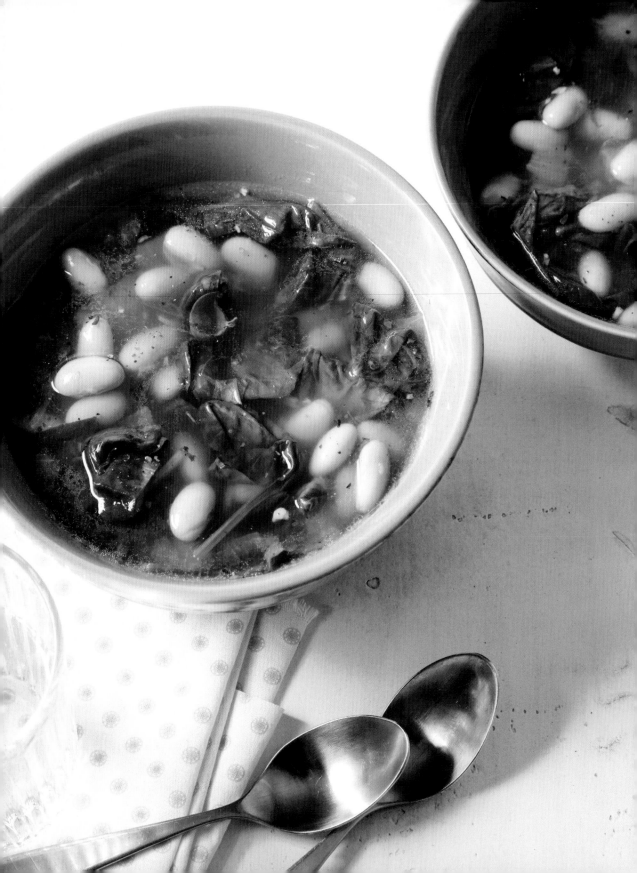

Garlic Spinach & White Bean Soup

Vegetable soup doesn't have to be boring!
This recipe is proof . . .

2 cups chopped onions
2 tablespoons whipped butter
1 tablespoon chopped garlic
5 cups roughly chopped spinach
4 cups low-sodium vegetable broth
One 15.5-ounce can cannellini (white kidney) beans, drained
   and rinsed
1 teaspoon onion powder
1 teaspoon salt
½ teaspoon dried oregano
½ teaspoon dried thyme

1. Bring a large pot sprayed with nonstick spray to
   medium-high heat. Add onions, butter, and garlic.
   Cook and stir until mostly softened, about 7 minutes.

2. Add remaining ingredients, and raise heat to high.
   Stirring occasionally, cook until onions are tender and
   soup is hot and well mixed, about 5 minutes.

MAKES 6 SERVINGS

121 calories

Prep: 10 minutes

Cook: 15 minutes

You'll need:
large pot,
nonstick spray

**⅙th of recipe
(about 1 cup):**
121 calories
2.5g total fat
(1g sat fat)
628mg sodium
19g carbs
5g fiber
4g sugars
5.5g protein

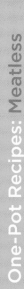

One-Pot Recipes: Meatless

Spicy Chickpea Chili

163 calories

1½ cups chopped brown mushrooms
1 cup chopped onion
1 cup chopped zucchini
One 14.5-ounce can crushed tomatoes
One 14.5-ounce can diced tomato with green chiles (not drained)
1 cup canned garbanzo beans, drained and rinsed
1 cup canned chili beans
2 teaspoons chopped garlic
1½ teaspoons chili powder
1 teaspoon ground cumin

1. Bring a large pot sprayed with nonstick spray to medium-high heat. Add mushrooms, onion, and zucchini. Cook and stir until softened, about 7 minutes.

2. Add remaining ingredients, and raise heat to high. Stirring occasionally, cook until veggies are tender and chili is hot and well mixed, about 4 minutes.

MAKES 5 SERVINGS

Prep: 10 minutes

Cook: 15 minutes

You'll need:
large pot,
nonstick spray

**⅕th of recipe
(about 1 cup):**
163 calories
1g total fat
(0g sat fat)
697mg sodium
29.5g carbs
8.5g fiber
8.5g sugars
8.5g protein

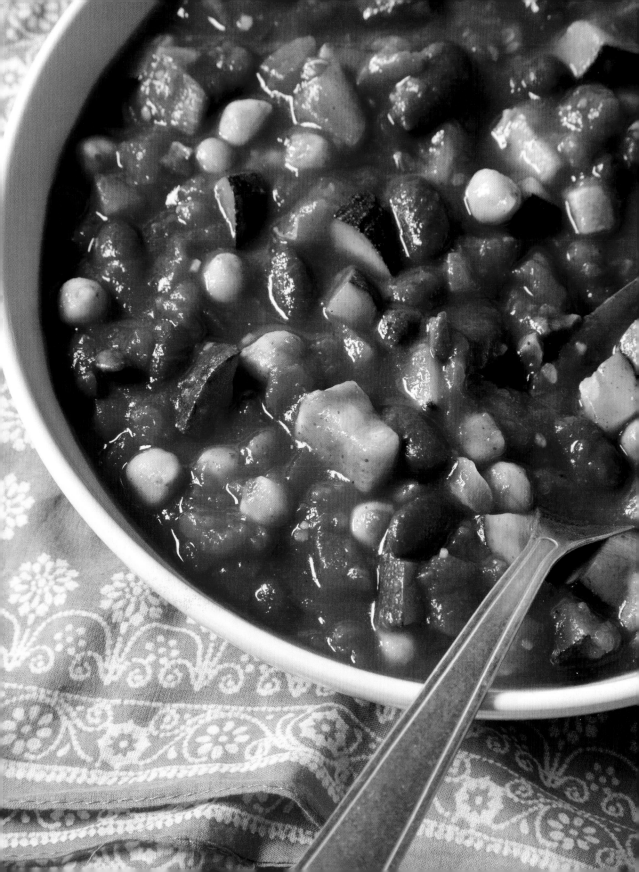

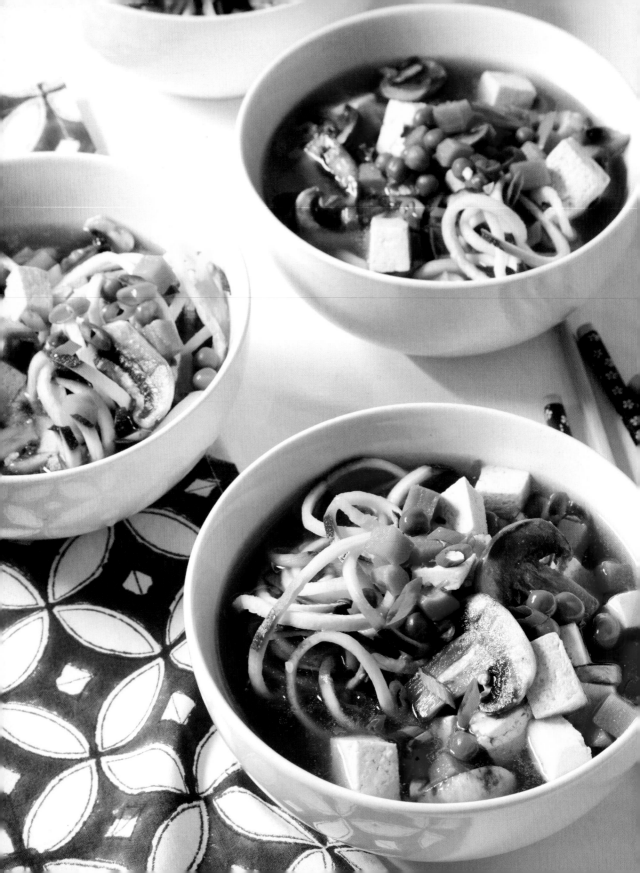

Zoodle Tofu Ramen

This soup is a total winner. You won't even miss the traditional noodles . . . promise!

1 pound (about 2 medium) spiralized zucchini, roughly chopped
2 cups thinly sliced mushrooms
4 cups vegetable broth
12 ounces block-style extra-firm tofu, excess moisture removed, cut into bite-size pieces
2 cups frozen peas and carrots, thawed
1 teaspoon garlic powder
1 teaspoon onion powder
½ teaspoon ground ginger
¼ teaspoon crushed red pepper
¼ cup chopped scallions

1. Bring a large pot sprayed with nonstick spray to medium-high heat. Add zucchini and mushrooms. Cook and stir until mostly softened, about 5 minutes.

2. Add broth, tofu, frozen veggies, and seasonings. Raise heat to high. Stirring occasionally, cook until veggies are tender and dish is hot and well mixed, about 6 minutes.

3. Serve topped with scallions.

MAKES 4 SERVINGS

30m V GF

179 calories

Prep: 10 minutes

Cook: 15 minutes

You'll need:
large pot,
nonstick spray

¼th of recipe (about 2 cups):
179 calories
5.5g total fat
(0.5g sat fat)
780mg sodium
17.5g carbs
5g fiber
9g sugars
14g protein

HG Tip
To save a little time, you can use frozen veggie spirals. Flip to page 314 for more on this subject!

One-Pot Recipes: Meatless

Hungry Girl FAST & Easy   239

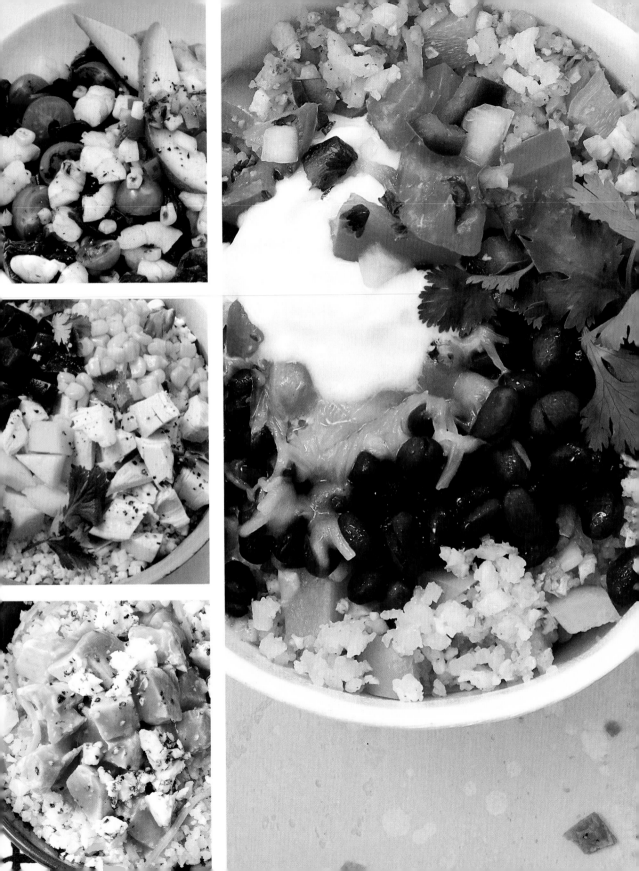

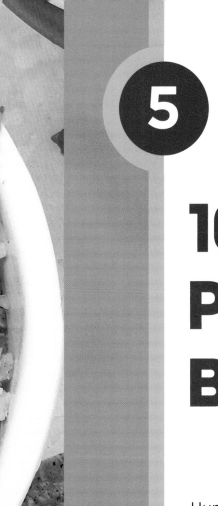

5

10-Minute Power Bowls

Hunger won't stand a chance against these protein-packed meals for one. They're great for last-minute lunches and dinners! Precooked protein is key here . . .

Creamy Pesto Chicken Bowl

2 tablespoons light/low-fat ricotta cheese
1 tablespoon pesto sauce
3 ounces cooked and chopped skinless chicken breast
1½ cups frozen riced cauliflower
¼ teaspoon garlic powder
¼ teaspoon onion powder
⅛ teaspoon salt
2 tablespoons chopped bagged sun-dried tomatoes (not packed in oil)
Optional topping: fresh basil

Prep: 5 minutes

Cook: 5 minutes

You'll need:
two medium microwave-safe bowls

Entire recipe:
319 calories
10.5g total fat
(2.5g sat fat)
575mg sodium
20.5g carbs
6.5g fiber
11g sugars
34.5g protein

1. In a medium microwave-safe bowl, mix ricotta with pesto until uniform. Add chicken, and stir to coat. Microwave for 30 seconds, or until hot.

2. Place cauliflower in a separate medium microwave-safe bowl. Microwave for 2 minutes, or until thawed and warm.

3. Mix garlic powder, onion powder, and salt into the cauliflower. Top with pesto chicken and tomatoes.

MAKES 1 SERVING

HG Tip
Like this? You'll love my one-pot Creamy Pesto Chicken on page 215!

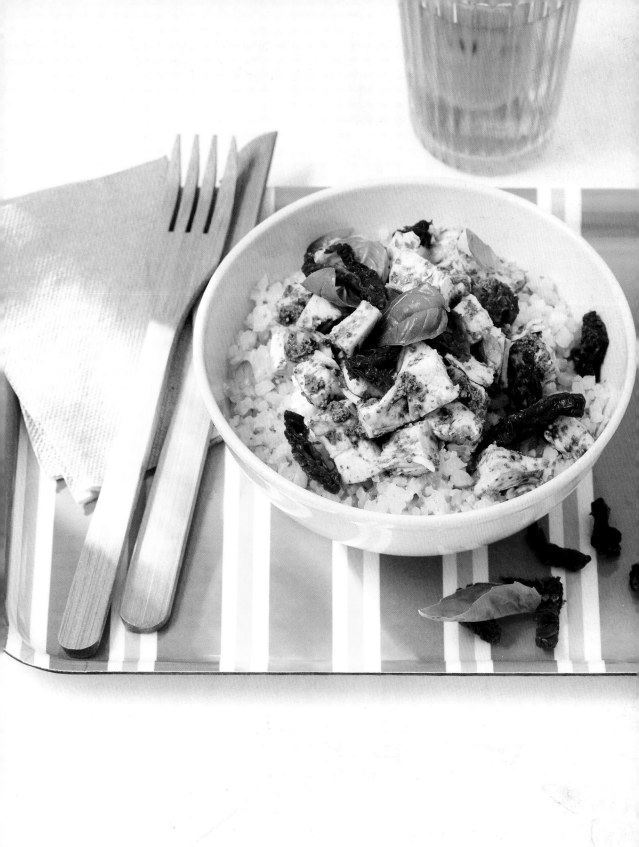

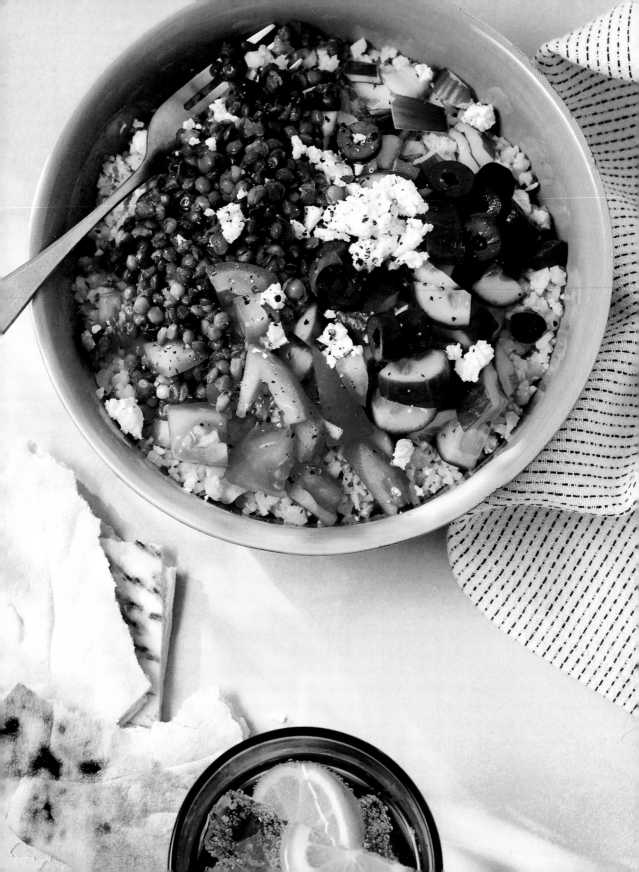

Greek Veggie Power Bowl

1½ cups frozen riced cauliflower
2 teaspoons light Italian dressing
⅛ teaspoon dried oregano
½ cup ready-to-eat lentils
⅓ cup chopped seedless cucumber
⅓ cup chopped tomato
2 tablespoons sliced Kalamata or black olives
2 tablespoons finely chopped red onion
2 tablespoons crumbled feta cheese

1. Place cauliflower in a medium microwave-safe bowl. Microwave for 2 minutes, or until thawed and warm.

2. Stir in Italian dressing and oregano. Top with remaining ingredients.

MAKES 1 SERVING

   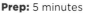

260 calories

Prep: 5 minutes

Cook: 5 minutes

You'll need:
medium microwave-safe bowl

Entire recipe:
260 calories
7.5g total fat
(2.5g sat fat)
735mg sodium
35.5g carbs
11.5g fiber
9g sugars
15g protein

HG FYI
Don't miss the Riced Cauliflower Guide on page 312!

Mango Chicken Power Bowl

266 calories

So fresh & fruity. This one's a keeper!

1½ cups frozen riced cauliflower
¼ teaspoon garlic powder
⅛ teaspoon salt
3 ounces cooked and chopped skinless chicken breast
¼ cup chopped mango
¼ cup drained and chopped canned beets
¼ cup frozen sweet corn kernels, thawed
1 tablespoon chopped fresh cilantro

1. Place cauliflower in a medium microwave-safe bowl. Cover and microwave for 2 minutes, or until thawed and warm.

2. Stir in garlic powder and salt. Top with remaining ingredients.

MAKES 1 SERVING

Prep: 5 minutes

Cook: 5 minutes

You'll need:
medium microwave-safe bowl

Entire recipe:
266 calories
4g total fat
(0.5g sat fat)
389mg sodium
27.5g carbs
6.5g fiber
15g sugars
31g protein

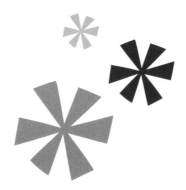

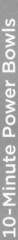
10-Minute Power Bowls

Hungry Girl FAST & Easy

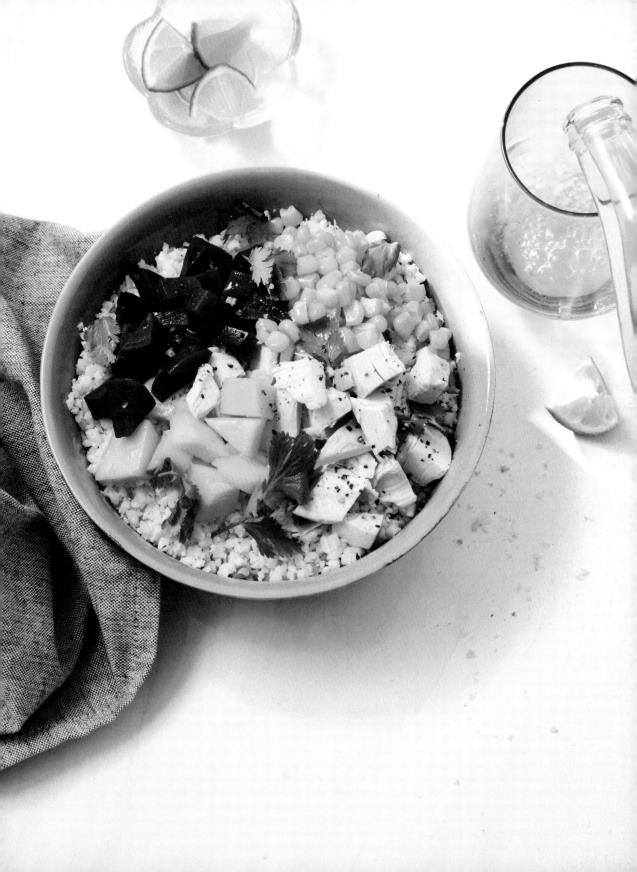

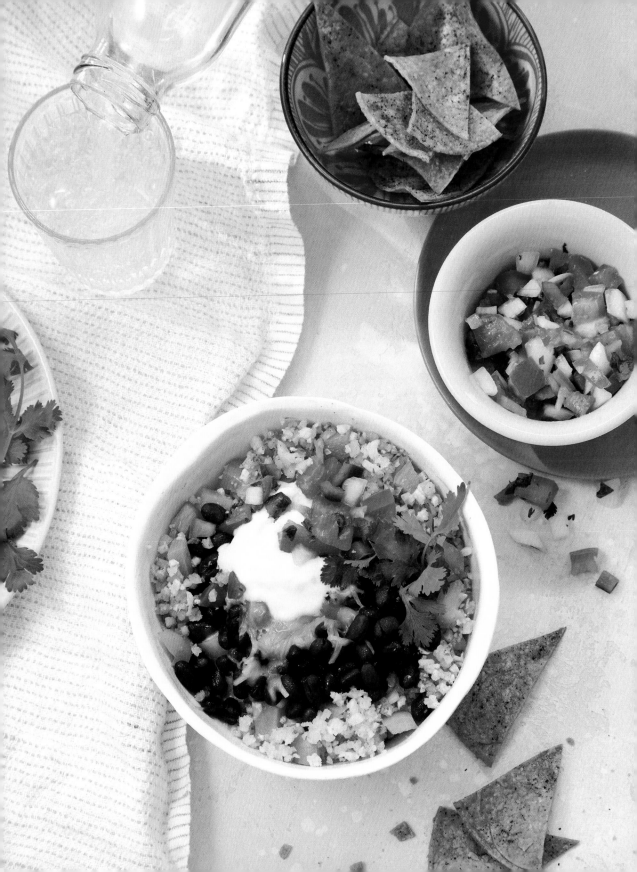

Meatless Burrito Bowl

1½ cups frozen riced cauliflower

½ cup chopped bell pepper

2 tablespoons chopped onion

1 teaspoon taco seasoning

2 teaspoons lime juice

⅓ cup canned black beans, drained and rinsed

2 tablespoons shredded reduced-fat Mexican-blend cheese

2 tablespoons salsa

1 tablespoon light sour cream

1 tablespoon chopped fresh cilantro

1. Place cauliflower, pepper, and onion in a medium microwave-safe bowl. Cover and microwave for 2 minutes, or until cauliflower has thawed and fresh veggies have softened.

2. Stir in taco seasoning and lime juice. Top with black beans and cheese, and microwave for 1 minute, or until hot.

3. Top with salsa, sour cream, and cilantro.

MAKES 1 SERVING

229 calories

Prep: 5 minutes

Cook: 5 minutes

You'll need:
medium microwave-safe bowl

Entire recipe:
229 calories
5g total fat
(2.5g sat fat)
700mg sodium
34.5g carbs
10g fiber
11.5g sugars
14g protein

10-Minute Power Bowls

Southwest Lentil Bowl

232 calories

5 cups spinach
½ cup ready-to-eat lentils
¼ cup black beans, drained and rinsed
¼ cup frozen sweet corn kernels, thawed
2 tablespoons salsa
1 tablespoon chopped fresh cilantro

1. Place spinach in a medium microwave-safe bowl. Microwave for 1 minute. Drain or blot away excess liquid.

2. Add lentils, black beans, and corn. Microwave for 1 more minute, or until hot.

3. Top with salsa and cilantro.

MAKES 1 SERVING

Prep: 5 minutes

Cook: 5 minutes

You'll need:
medium microwave-safe bowl

Entire recipe:
232 calories
1g total fat
(0g sat fat)
650mg sodium
42.5g carbs
13g fiber
6.5g sugars
16.5g protein

HG Tip
Look for cooked lentils in the produce section or with the canned food.

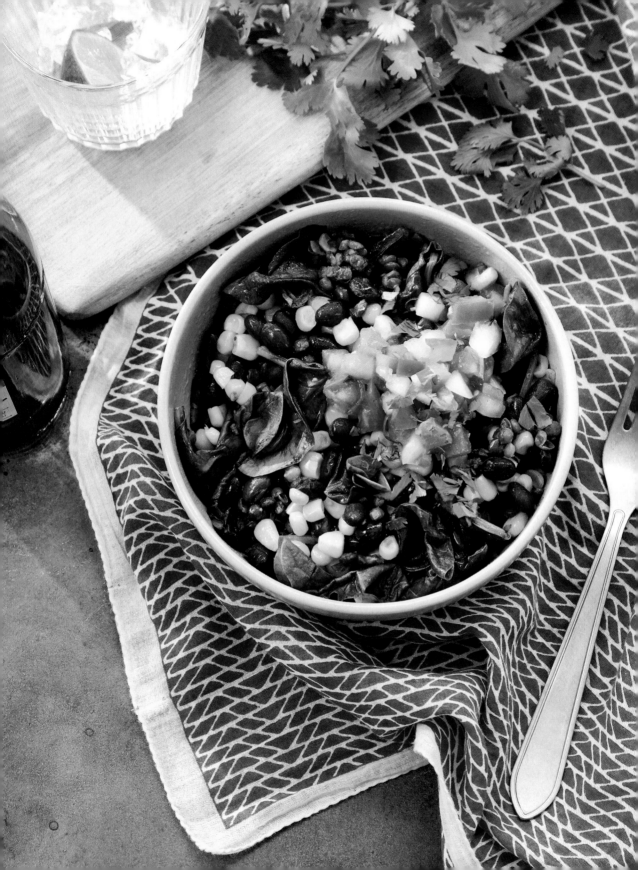

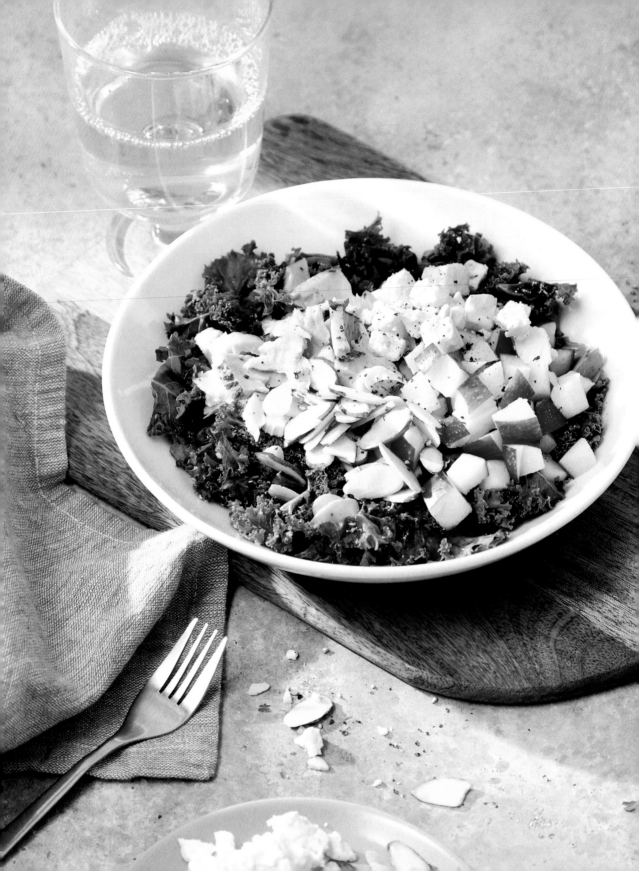

Kale, Turkey & Apple Power Bowl

The first time I made this, something was missing . . . Feta made it betta'!

3 cups chopped kale

1 tablespoon light balsamic vinaigrette

2 ounces (about 4 slices) reduced-sodium skinless turkey breast, roughly chopped

½ cup chopped Fuji or Gala apple

¼ ounce (about 1 tablespoon) sliced almonds

1½ tablespoons crumbled feta cheese

1. Place kale in a medium microwave-safe bowl. Add 2 tablespoons water, cover, and microwave for 2 minutes, or until softened. Drain or blot away excess liquid.

2. Add vinaigrette, and stir. Top with turkey, apple, almonds, and feta.

MAKES 1 SERVING

15m GF

212 calories

Prep: 5 minutes

Cook: 5 minutes

You'll need:
medium microwave-safe bowl

Entire recipe:
212 calories
8.5g total fat
(2g sat fat)
607mg sodium
17g carbs
4.5g fiber
9g sugars
18.5g protein

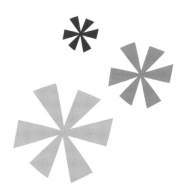

Shrimp & Blackened Corn Power Bowl

Shrimp and corn are quite the power couple! (They also team up on page 231 for my Shrimp & Bacon Corn Chowder.)

Prep: 5 minutes

Cook: 5 minutes

You'll need:
medium microwave-safe bowl, skillet, nonstick spray

Entire recipe:
231 calories
6.5g total fat
(1g sat fat)
625mg sodium
20.5g carbs
6.5g fiber
6g sugars
26.5g protein

5 cups spinach
¼ teaspoon garlic powder
Dash salt
¼ cup frozen sweet corn kernels, thawed
½ cup cherry tomatoes, halved
3 ounces (about 6 large) ready-to-eat shrimp, chopped
1 ounce (about ¼ cup) sliced avocado
2 tablespoons salsa

1. Place spinach in a medium microwave-safe bowl. Microwave for 1 minute. Drain or blot away excess liquid. Sprinkle with garlic powder and salt.

2. Bring a skillet sprayed with nonstick spray to high heat. Add corn. Cook and stir until blackened, about 3 minutes. Add tomatoes, and cook until hot and blackened, about 1 minute.

3. Remove from heat, and stir in shrimp. Spoon mixture over the spinach, and top with avocado and salsa.

MAKES 1 SERVING

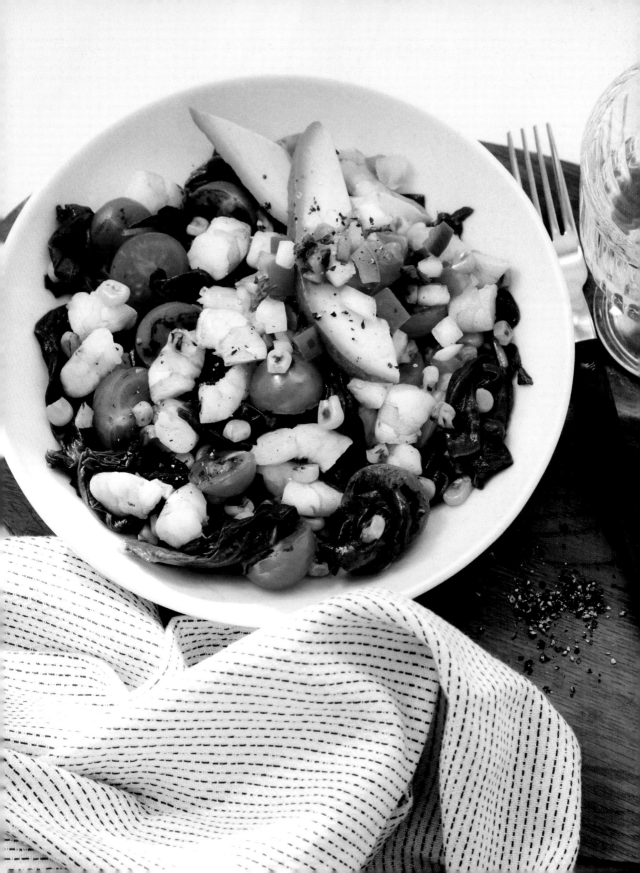

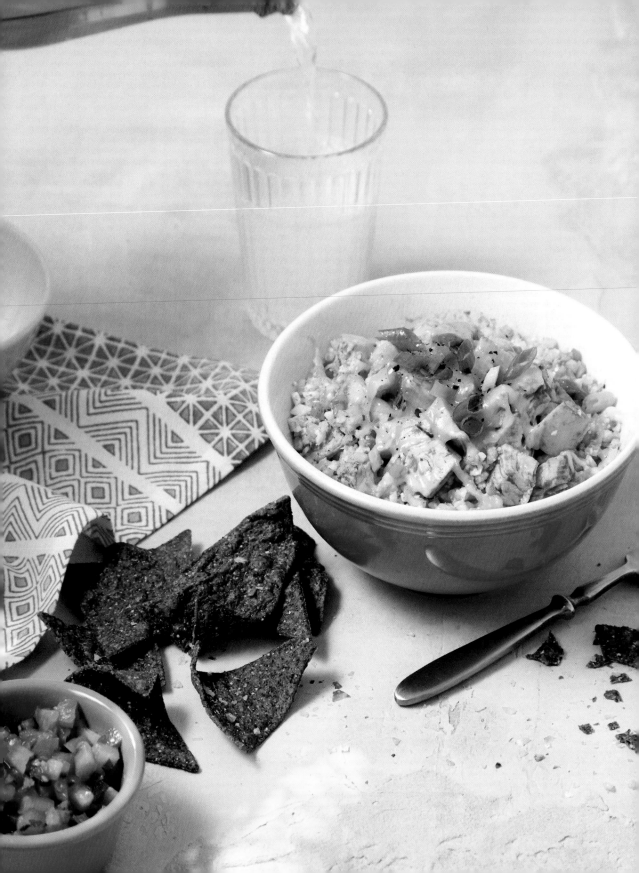

Chicken Enchilada Bowl

1½ cups frozen riced cauliflower
¼ cup finely chopped onion
1 teaspoon taco seasoning
3 ounces cooked and chopped skinless chicken breast
2 tablespoons red enchilada sauce
2 tablespoons shredded reduced-fat Mexican-blend cheese
Optional topping: scallions

1. Place cauliflower and onion in a medium microwave-safe bowl. Microwave for 2 minutes, or until cauliflower has thawed and onion has softened. Stir in taco seasoning.

2. In a separate medium bowl, coat chicken with enchilada sauce. Spoon over veggies, and top with cheese. Microwave for 1½ minutes, or until chicken is hot and cheese has melted.

MAKES 1 SERVING

Prep: 5 minutes

Cook: 5 minutes

You'll need:
medium microwave-safe bowl, medium bowl

Entire recipe:
280 calories
7g total fat
(2.5g sat fat)
511mg sodium
20.5g carbs
6g fiber
8g sugars
34.5g protein

280 calories

Asian-Style Shrimp & Zucchini Noodle Bowl

280 calories

8 ounces (about 1 medium) spiralized zucchini, roughly chopped

3 ounces (about 6 large) ready-to-eat shrimp, chopped

3 tablespoons Thai peanut sauce/salad dressing with 65 calories or less per 2-tablespoon serving

2 tablespoons canned sliced water chestnuts, drained and chopped

2 tablespoons chopped scallions

¼ ounce (about 1 tablespoon) crushed peanuts

 15m

Prep: 5 minutes

Cook: 5 minutes

You'll need:
skillet, nonstick spray, strainer, medium bowl

Entire recipe:
280 calories
10g total fat
(1g sat fat)
716mg sodium
22g carbs
4g fiber
15.5g sugars
27.5g protein

1. Bring a skillet sprayed with nonstick spray to medium-high heat. Add zucchini, and cook and stir until hot and slightly softened, about 3 minutes.

2. Add shrimp, and cook and stir until hot, about 1 minute. Transfer to a strainer, and thoroughly drain excess liquid.

3. Transfer zucchini and shrimp to a medium bowl. Add peanut sauce/dressing, and stir to coat. Top with water chestnuts, scallions, and peanuts.

MAKES 1 SERVING

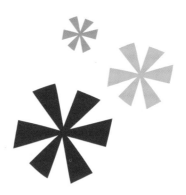

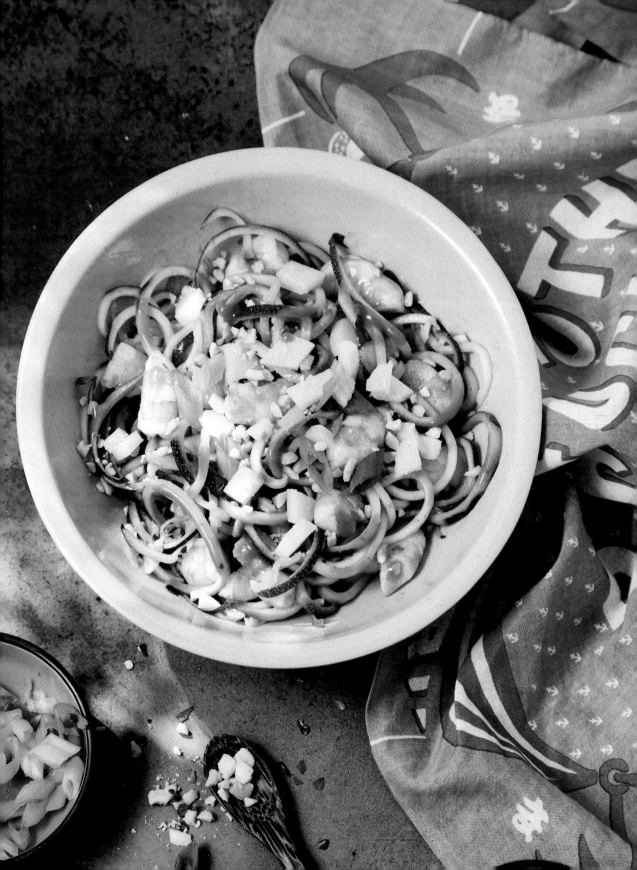

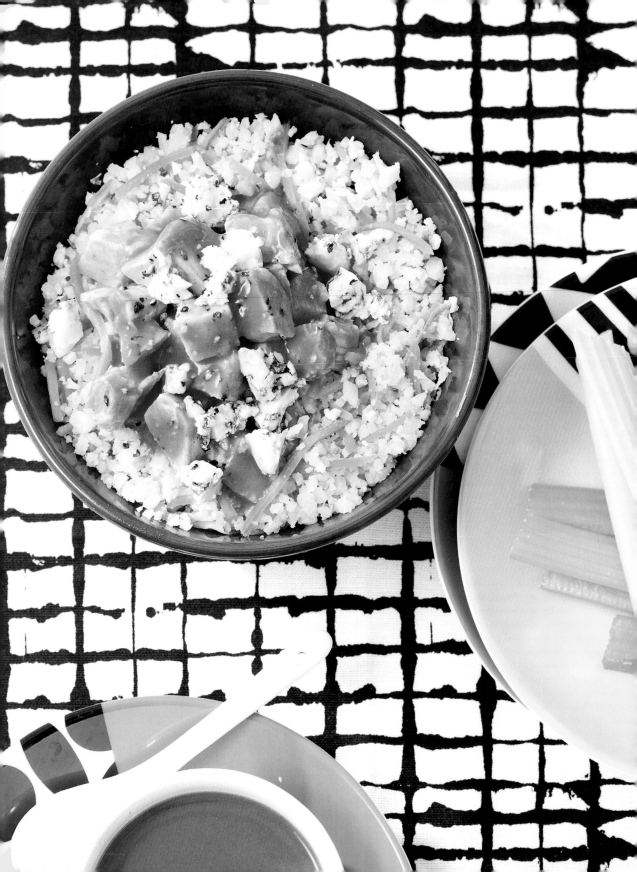

Buffalo Chicken Power Bowl

This one tastes just like hot wings with blue cheese dressing. (In fairness, anything tastes like hot wings when you douse it in Frank's!)

1¼ cups frozen riced cauliflower
¼ cup shredded carrots
¼ teaspoon garlic powder
¼ teaspoon onion powder
3 ounces cooked and chopped skinless chicken breast
1 tablespoon Frank's RedHot Original Cayenne Pepper Sauce, or more for topping
1½ tablespoons crumbled blue cheese

1. Place cauliflower and carrots in a medium microwave-safe bowl. Cover and microwave for 2 minutes, or until cauliflower has thawed, carrots have softened, and both veggies are hot. Stir in garlic powder and onion powder.

2. In a separate medium microwave-safe bowl, coat chicken with hot sauce. Microwave for 30 seconds, or until hot. Spoon over veggie bowl, and top with blue cheese.

MAKES 1 SERVING

236 calories

Prep: 5 minutes

Cook: 5 minutes

You'll need:
two medium microwave-safe bowls

Entire recipe:
236 calories
6.5g total fat
(2.5g sat fat)
832mg sodium
12g carbs
4.5g fiber
5.5g sugars
32g protein

10-Minute Power Bowls

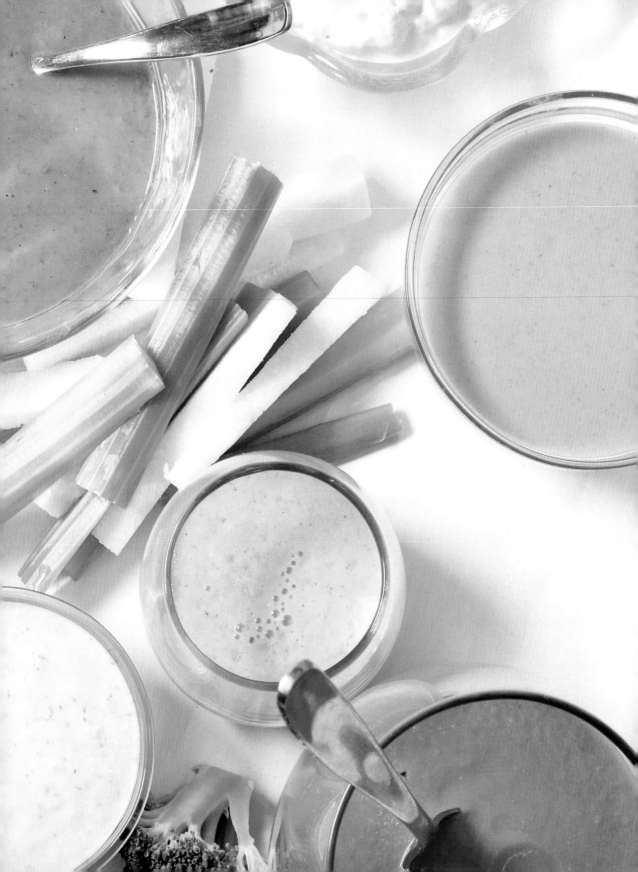

6

5-Minute Salad Dressings

Dressing can make or break a salad, and these simple creations are next level. My personal favorite? The Everything Bagel Dressing, page 266!

HG FYI
Store your dressing in a medium sealable container in the fridge. It'll stay fresh for about two weeks!

Roasted Red Pepper Dressing

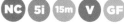

22 calories

NC 5i 15m V GF

⅛th of recipe (about 2 tablespoons): 22 calories, 0g total fat (0g sat fat), 121mg sodium, 4.5g carbs, 0g fiber, 4g sugars, 0.5g protein

¾ cup roasted red peppers packed in water, drained
¼ cup fat-free plain Greek yogurt
3 tablespoons apple cider vinegar
1 tablespoon honey
½ teaspoon ground cumin
¼ teaspoon salt

HG Tip
Use a food processor or small blender like the NutriBullet for this and other blended dressings. It's the perfect size and so easy to use!

Blend ingredients until smooth and uniform.

MAKES 8 SERVINGS

Creamy Balsamic Vinaigrette

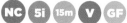

57 calories

NC 5i 15m V GF

⅛th of recipe (about 2 tablespoons): 57 calories, 3.5g total fat (0.5g sat fat), 191mg sodium, 4.5g carbs, 0g fiber, 4g sugars, 1.5g protein

½ cup fat-free plain Greek yogurt
⅓ cup balsamic vinegar
2 tablespoons olive oil
1 tablespoon Dijon mustard
1 tablespoon honey
½ teaspoon garlic powder
½ teaspoon onion powder
½ teaspoon salt
¼ teaspoon black pepper

Blend ingredients until smooth and uniform.

MAKES 8 SERVINGS

5-Minute Salad Dressings

Creamy Salsa Dressing

    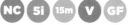

13 calories

⅛th of recipe (about 2 tablespoons): 13 calories, 0g total fat (0g sat fat), 142mg sodium, 2g carbs, 0g fiber, 1.5g sugars, 1g protein

⅔ **cup salsa**
⅓ **cup fat-free plain Greek yogurt**
2 **teaspoons lime juice**
1 **teaspoon taco seasoning**

Combine ⅓ cup salsa with remaining ingredients, and blend until smooth and uniform. Stir in remaining ⅓ cup salsa.

MAKES 8 SERVINGS

Asian-Style Peanut Dressing

61 calories

⅛th of recipe (about 2 tablespoons): 61 calories, 3g total fat (0.5g sat fat), 259mg sodium, 5g carbs, 1g fiber, 2g sugars, 4.5g protein

½ **cup powdered peanut butter**
¼ **cup unsweetened plain almond milk**
2 **tablespoons creamy peanut butter**
2 **tablespoons seasoned rice vinegar**
2 **tablespoons reduced-sodium/lite soy sauce**
1 **teaspoon lime juice**
1 **teaspoon dried minced onion**
½ **teaspoon garlic powder**
¼ **teaspoon cayenne pepper**

Mix ingredients until smooth and uniform.

MAKES 8 SERVINGS

5-Minute Salad Dressings

Honey Mustard Dressing

56 calories

   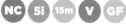

⅛th of recipe (about 2 tablespoons): 56 calories, 0g total fat (0g sat fat), 460mg sodium, 9.5g carbs, 0g fiber, 9g sugars, 0g protein

¾ cup Dijon mustard
¼ cup honey
1½ tablespoons apple cider vinegar

Combine ingredients with ¼ cup water, and mix until smooth and uniform.

MAKES 8 SERVINGS

Everything Bagel Dressing

59 calories

   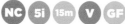

⅛th of recipe (about 2 tablespoons): 59 calories, 4g total fat (2.5g sat fat), 176mg sodium, 2.5g carbs, 2g sugars, 1.5g protein

½ cup light/reduced-fat cream cheese
½ cup light sour cream
1 teaspoon Dijon mustard
½ teaspoon lemon juice
½ teaspoon garlic powder
2 teaspoons everything bagel seasoning

Combine all ingredients except bagel seasoning with 2 teaspoons water, and blend until smooth and uniform. Stir in bagel seasoning.

MAKES 8 SERVINGS

5-Minute Salad Dressings

Carrot Ginger Dressing

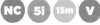

35
calories

⅛th of recipe (about 2 tablespoons): 35 calories, 1.5g total fat (<0.5g sat fat), 265mg sodium, 4.5g carbs, <0.5g fiber, 3.5g sugars, <0.5g protein

¾ **cup pureed carrots (found in the baby food aisle)**
¼ **cup seasoned rice vinegar**
1 tablespoon sesame oil
1 tablespoon reduced-sodium/lite soy sauce
1 teaspoon ground ginger

Mix ingredients until smooth and uniform.

MAKES 8 SERVINGS

Avocado Lime Dressing

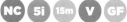

30
calories

⅛th of recipe (about 2 tablespoons): 30 calories, 2g total fat (<0.5g sat fat), 78mg sodium, 2g carbs, 1g fiber, 0.5g sugars, 1g protein

4 ounces (about ½ cup) chopped avocado
½ **cup fresh cilantro**
¼ **cup fat-free plain Greek yogurt**
2 tablespoons lime juice
1 teaspoon ground cumin
½ **teaspoon garlic powder**
¼ **teaspoon salt**

Combine ingredients with ½ cup water, and blend until smooth and uniform.

MAKES 8 SERVINGS

5-Minute Salad Dressings

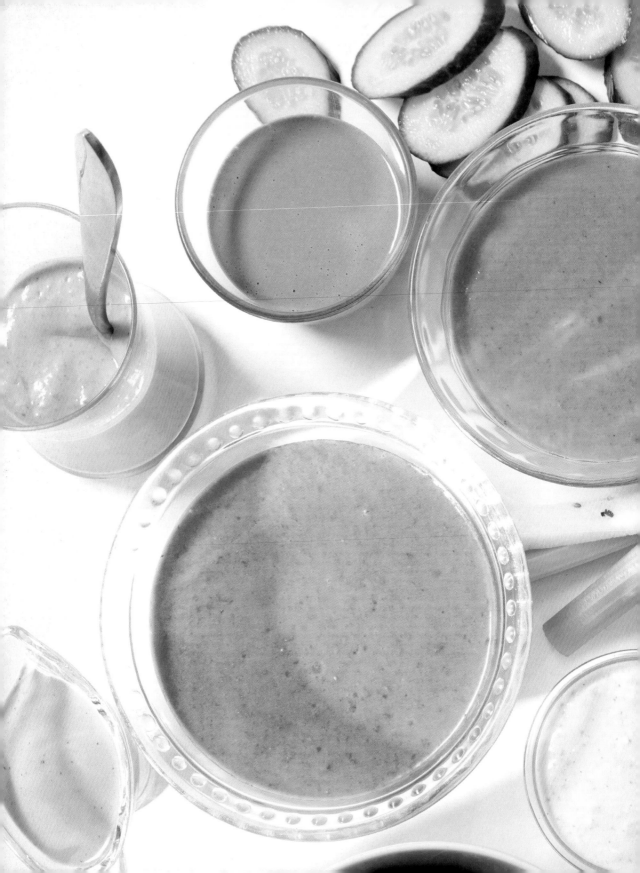

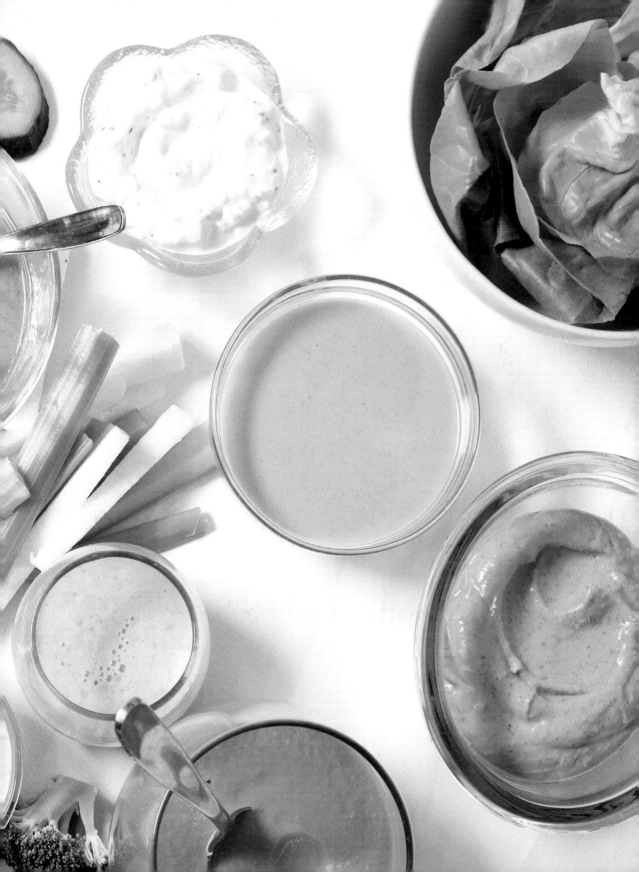

Raspberry Vinaigrette

59 calories

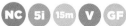

⅛th of recipe (about 2 tablespoons): 59 calories, 5g total fat (0.5g sat fat), 37mg sodium, 3g carbs, 1g fiber, 1g sugars, <0.5g protein

1 cup raspberries (fresh or thawed from frozen)
¼ cup lemon juice
¼ cup red wine vinegar
3 tablespoons olive oil
5 packets natural no-calorie sweetener
⅛ teaspoon salt

Blend ingredients until smooth and uniform.

MAKES 8 SERVINGS

Green Goddess Dressing

29 calories

⅛th of recipe (about 2 tablespoons): 29 calories, 2g total fat (<0.5g sat fat), 151mg sodium, 1.5g carbs, 0.5g fiber, 0.5g sugars, 1g protein

½ cup chopped parsley
¼ cup fat-free plain Greek yogurt
¼ cup chopped scallions
1 ounce (about 2 tablespoons) chopped avocado
2 tablespoons lemon juice
1 tablespoon olive oil
2 teaspoons chopped garlic
½ teaspoon salt

Combine ingredients with ¼ cup water, and blend until smooth and uniform.

MAKES 8 SERVINGS

5-Minute Salad Dressings

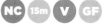

33 calories

⅛th of recipe (about 2 tablespoons): 33 calories, 1.5g total fat (1g sat fat), 167mg sodium, 1.5g carbs, 0g fiber, 1g sugars, 3.5g protein

½ cup crumbled feta cheese
¾ cup fat-free plain Greek yogurt
¼ cup chopped and seeded cucumber, patted dry
2 tablespoons chopped fresh dill
1 tablespoon white wine vinegar
1 teaspoon chopped garlic
¼ teaspoon salt

Combine ¼ cup feta with remaining ingredients, and blend until smooth and uniform. Stir in remaining ¼ cup feta.

MAKES 8 SERVINGS

5-Minute Salad Dressings

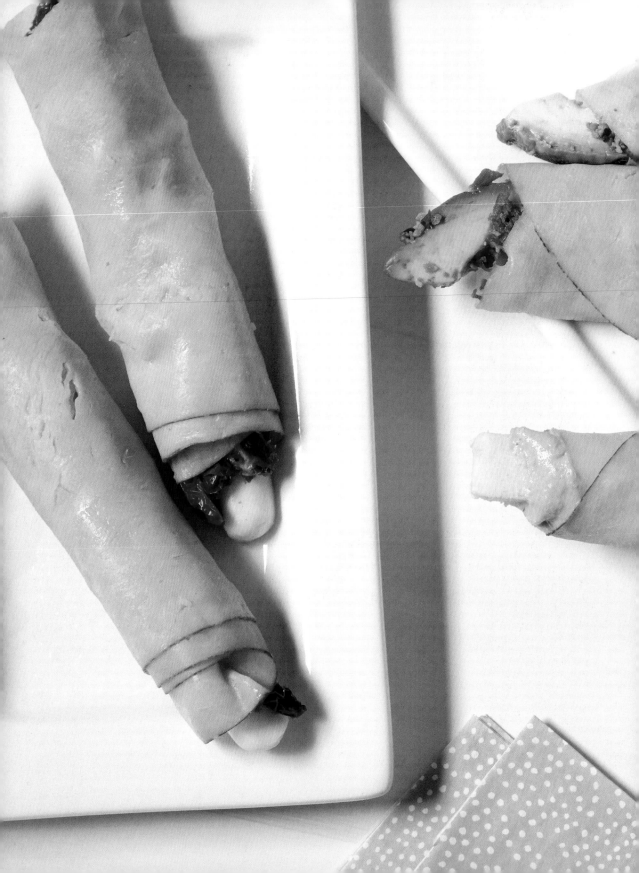

7

3-Ingredient Protein Rollups

These quickie creations are go-to snacks for me. So satisfying, no cooking necessary, and ready in five minutes!

Turkey, Hummus & Jicama Rollups

   GF

Entire recipe (2 rollups): 128 calories, 5g total fat (0.5g sat fat), 440mg sodium, 6.5g carbs, 2g fiber, 1g sugars, 14g protein

2 tablespoons hummus
4 slices (about 2 ounces) reduced-sodium skinless turkey breast
4 jicama spears

Spread half of the hummus over 2 turkey slices, top with 2 jicama spears, and roll it up. Repeat with remaining ingredients.

MAKES 1 SERVING

Ham, Swiss & Cucumber Rollups

    GF

Entire recipe (2 rollups): 133 calories, 5g total fat (2g sat fat), 507mg sodium, 4.5g carbs, 0.5g fiber, 2.5g sugar, 16.5g protein

2 slices (about 2 ounces) reduced-sodium ham
1 slice reduced-fat Swiss cheese, halved
2 cucumber spears

Top each ham slice with half a cheese slice and 1 cucumber spear, and roll it up.

MAKES 1 SERVING

Turkey, Avocado & Bacon Rollups

127 calories

Entire recipe (2 rollups): 127 calories, 6g total fat (1.5g sat fat), 505mg sodium, 2.5g carbs, 2g fiber, <0.5g sugars, 15g protein

1 ounce (about ¼ cup) sliced avocado
4 slices (about 2 ounces) reduced-sodium skinless turkey breast
1 tablespoon precooked crumbled bacon

Spread half of the avocado over 2 turkey slices, top with half of the bacon, and roll it up. Repeat with remaining ingredients.

MAKES 1 SERVING

Roast Beef, Cheddar & Pickle Rollups

157 calories

Entire recipe (2 rollups): 157 calories, 7g total fat (3.5g sat fat), 489mg sodium, 1.5g carbs, 0.5g fiber, 0.5g sugars, 21g protein

4 slices (about 2 ounces) low-sodium roast beef
1 slice reduced-fat cheddar cheese, halved
6 dill pickle chips

Top 2 roast beef slices with half a cheese slice and 3 pickle chips, and roll it up. Repeat with remaining ingredients.

MAKES 1 SERVING

3-Ingredient Protein Rollups

Turkey, String Cheese & Tomato Rollups

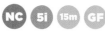 NC 5i 15m GF

Entire recipe (2 rollups): 154 calories, 3.5g total fat (1.5g sat fat), 528mg sodium, 8.5g carbs, 2g fiber, 4.5g sugars, 20.5g protein

4 slices (about 2 ounces) reduced-sodium skinless turkey breast
1 stick light string cheese, halved
2 tablespoons bagged sun-dried tomatoes (not packed in oil)

Top 2 turkey slices with half a cheese stick and half of the tomatoes, and roll it up. Repeat with remaining ingredients.

MAKES 1 SERVING

 Make It Vegan . . .
Swap the meat & cheese for vegan deli slices and dairy-free cheese. Flip to page 320 for more vegan swaps!

3-Ingredient Protein Rollups

Hungry Girl *FAST* & Easy

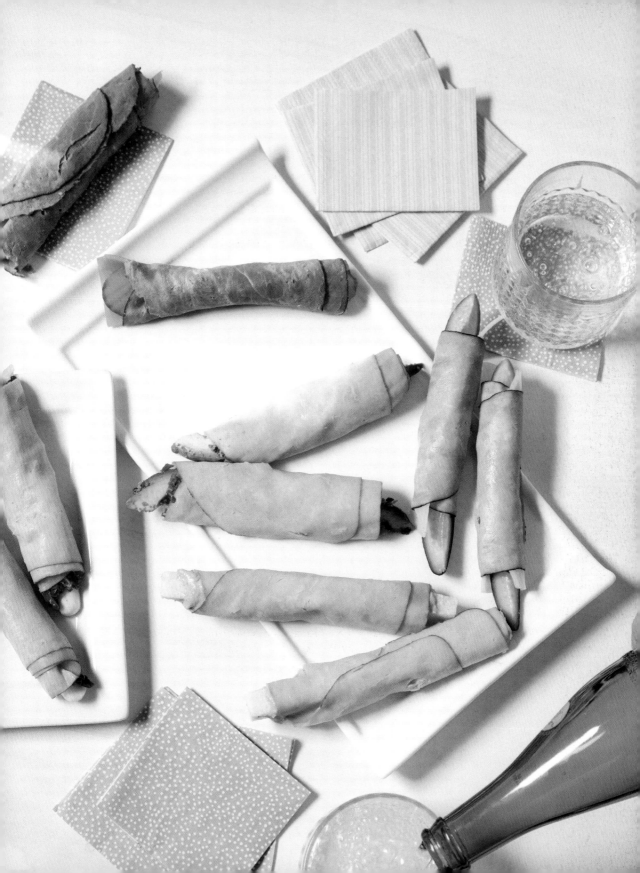

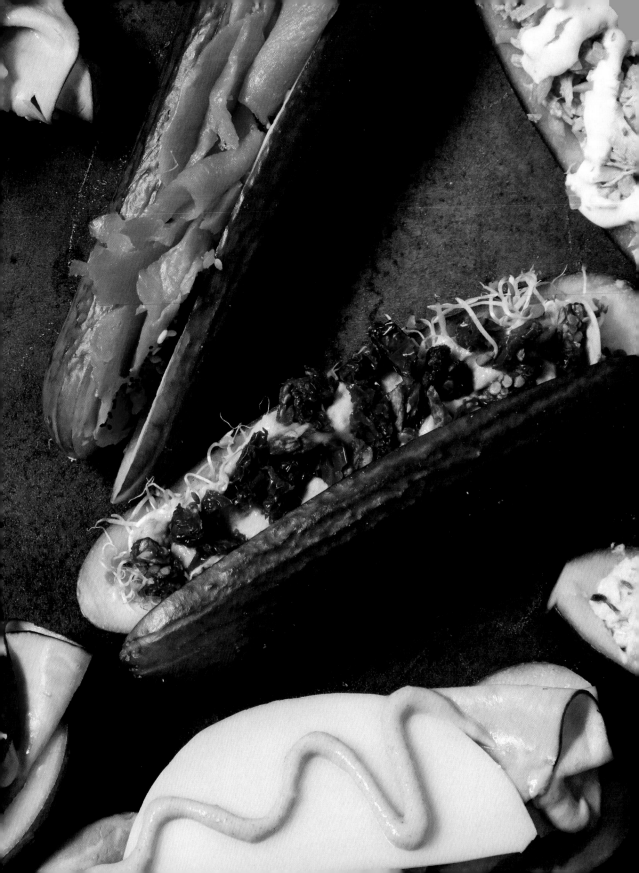

8

Speedy Cucumber Subs

Ditch the carbs and make sandwich buns out of cucumbers! These recipes are perfect for snacks, meals . . . even party platters. Look for the to ID the ones that also work with the pickle of your choice in place of the cucumber!

How to Make Cucumber Subs

Slice off and discard stem ends of two small (about 5-ounce) cucumbers. Halve cucumbers lengthwise. Gently scoop out and discard the cucumber flesh, leaving about ¼ inch inside each half. Thoroughly pat dry.

Club Sandwich Cucumber Subs

200 calories

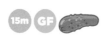

Entire recipe (2 subs): 200 calories, 10g total fat (2g sat fat), 782mg sodium, 9.5g carbs, 2.5g fiber, 5.5g sugars, 17.5g protein

2 slices center-cut bacon or turkey bacon
1 ounce (about 2 slices) reduced-sodium ham
1 ounce (about 2 slices) reduced-sodium skinless turkey breast
1 tablespoon light mayonnaise
4 small tomato slices
2 cucumber subs (4 halves)

Cook bacon until crispy, and layer with remaining ingredients between cucumber subs.

MAKES 1 SERVING

Speedy Cucumber Subs

Veggie Lovers Cucumber Subs

  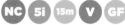

130 calories

Entire recipe (2 subs): 130 calories, 4.5g total fat (0.5g sat fat), 156mg sodium, 16.5g carbs, 4.5g fiber, 8g sugars, 4.5g protein

¼ cup alfalfa sprouts
2 tablespoons hummus
2 tablespoons bagged sun-dried tomatoes (not packed in oil)
2 cucumber subs (4 halves)

Layer ingredients between cucumber subs.

MAKES 1 SERVING

Lox & Cream Cheese Cucumber Subs

   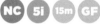

165 calories

Entire recipe (2 subs): 165 calories, 8.5g total fat (4g sat fat), 818mg sodium, 6.5g carbs, 1.5g fiber, 4.5g sugars, 14g protein

2 tablespoons light/reduced-fat cream cheese
2 ounces smoked salmon with 300mg sodium or less per ounce
¼ teaspoon everything bagel seasoning
2 cucumber subs (4 halves)

Layer ingredients between cucumber subs.

MAKES 1 SERVING

Speedy Cucumber Subs

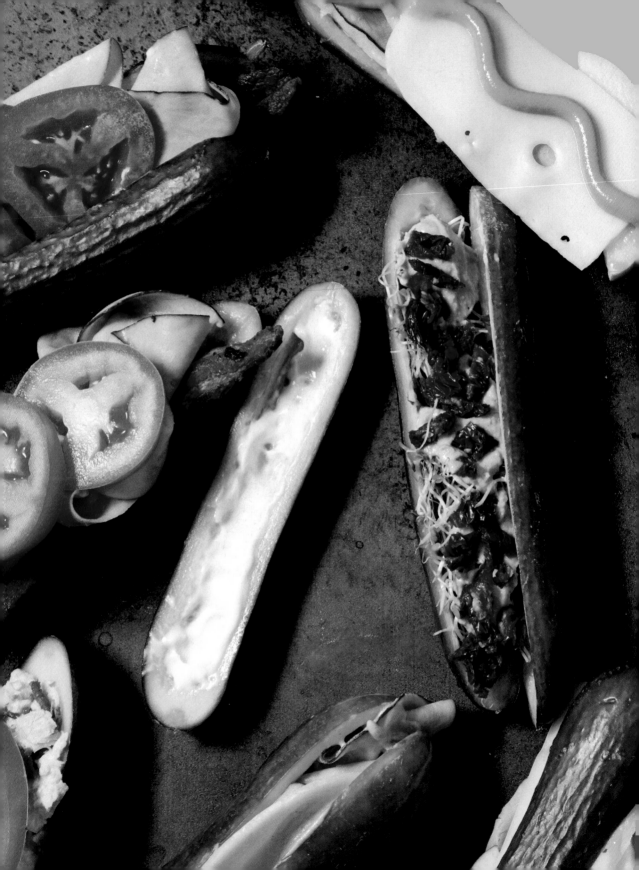

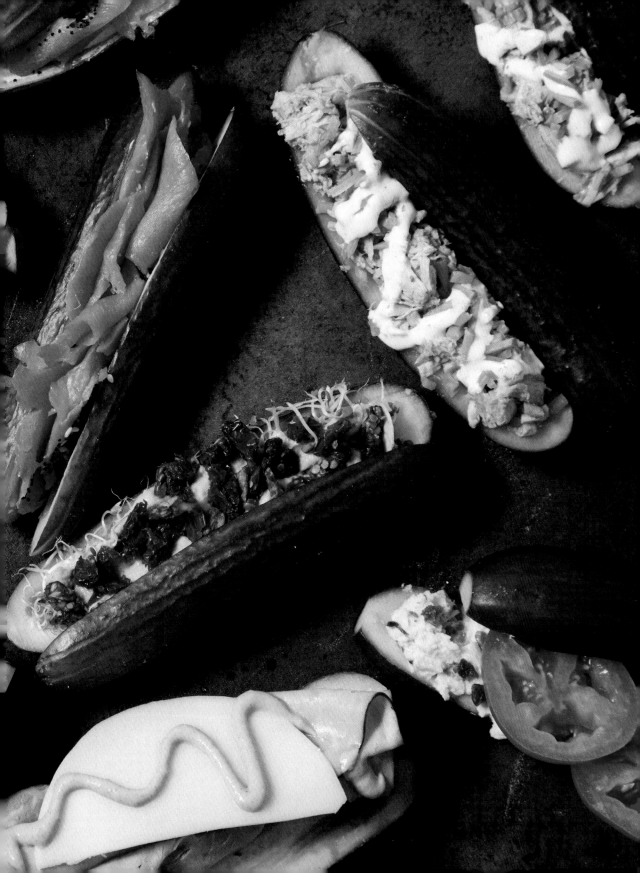

Ham, Apple & Swiss Cucumber Subs

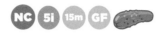

188 calories

NC 5i 15m GF

Entire recipe (2 subs): 188 calories, 5.5g total fat (2.5g sat fat), 605mg sodium, 15g carbs, 2.5g fiber, 10.5g sugars, 17.5g protein

2 ounces (about 4 slices) reduced-sodium ham
4 thin apple slices
1 slice reduced-fat Swiss cheese, halved
2 teaspoons honey mustard
2 cucumber subs (4 halves)

Layer ingredients between cucumber subs.

MAKES 1 SERVING

Ranch & Bacon Tuna Cucumber Subs

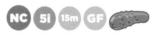

181 calories

NC 5i 15m GF

Entire recipe (2 subs): 181 calories, 7g total fat (1.5g sat fat), 532mg sodium, 8g carbs, 2.5g fiber, 5.5g sugars, 20.5g protein

One 2.6-ounce pouch albacore tuna packed in water, flaked
1 tablespoon light ranch dressing
4 small tomato slices
1 tablespoon precooked crumbled bacon
2 cucumber subs (4 halves)

Combine tuna with dressing, and layer with remaining ingredients between cucumber subs.

MAKES 1 SERVING

Speedy Cucumber Subs

Hungry Girl FAST & Easy

Ham & Provolone Cucumber Subs

   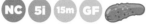

Entire recipe (2 subs): 147 calories, 5.5g total fat (2.5g sat fat), 733mg sodium, 6.5g carbs, 1.5g fiber, 4g sugars, 16.5g protein

2 ounces (about 4 slices) reduced-sodium ham
1 slice reduced-fat provolone cheese, halved
2 teaspoons Dijon mustard
2 cucumber subs (4 halves)

Layer ingredients between cucumber subs.

MAKES 1 SERVING

Buffalo Chicken Cucumber Subs

   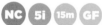

Entire recipe (2 subs): 149 calories, 4.5g total fat (0.5g sat fat), 522mg sodium, 6.5g carbs, 2g fiber, 4.5g sugars, 19g protein

2 ounces cooked and shredded skinless chicken breast
2 teaspoons Frank's RedHot Original Cayenne Pepper Sauce
2 tablespoons shredded carrots, chopped
2 teaspoons light ranch dressing
2 cucumber subs (4 halves)

Mix chicken with hot sauce, and layer with remaining ingredients between cucumber subs.

MAKES 1 SERVING

HG Tip
Buffalo chicken fans . . . Don't miss the Buffalo Chicken Power Bowl on page 261!

Speedy Cucumber Subs

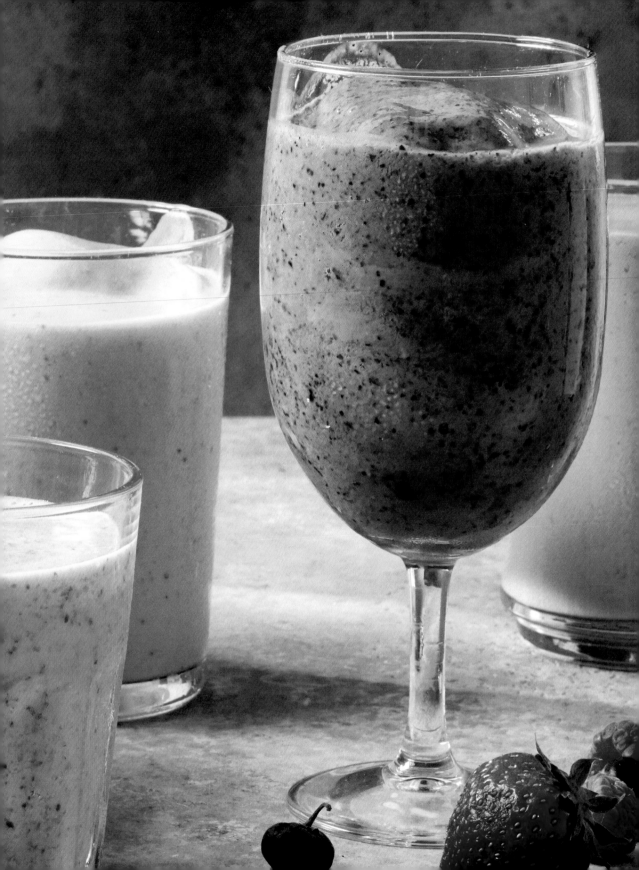

9

5-Minute Smoothies

These aren't your average blended beverages . . . Each one starts with a single-serve container of Greek yogurt, delivering a protein punch! Grab your blender, and put these combos into regular rotation.

HG Tip
Buying yogurt in bulk containers? You'll need ½ cup for each of these smoothies.

Strawberry Banana Smoothie

  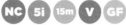

Entire recipe (about 14 ounces): 216 calories, 2g total fat (0g sat fat), 153mg sodium, 34.5g carbs, 4.5g fiber, 20.5g sugars, 17.5g protein

¾ cup frozen strawberries
½ cup frozen banana coins
½ cup unsweetened vanilla almond milk
One 5.3-ounce container fat-free plain Greek yogurt
2 packets natural no-calorie sweetener, or more to taste

Blend ingredients until smooth.

MAKES 1 SERVING

Grapes & Greens Smoothie

224 calories

  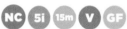

Entire recipe (about 18 ounces): 224 calories, 1.5g total fat (0g sat fat), 178mg sodium, 37g carbs, 2g fiber, 29.5g sugars, 17.5g protein

1 cup frozen green grapes
1 cup spinach leaves
½ cup unsweetened vanilla almond milk
One 5.3-ounce container fat-free plain Greek yogurt
2 packets natural no-calorie sweetener, or more to taste
½ cup crushed ice

Blend ingredients until smooth.

MAKES 1 SERVING

5-Minute Smoothies

Hungry Girl FAST & Easy

Peanut Butter Apple Smoothie

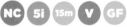

224 calories

Entire recipe (about 20 ounces): 224 calories, 3.5g total fat, (<0.5g sat fat), 185mg sodium, 28.5g carbs, 4g fiber, 19.5g sugars, 22.5g protein

1 cup chopped Fuji apple
½ cup unsweetened vanilla almond milk
One 5.3-ounce container fat-free plain Greek yogurt
2 tablespoons powdered peanut butter
2 packets natural no-calorie sweetener, or more to taste
1–1½ cups crushed ice

Blend ingredients until smooth.

MAKES 1 SERVING

Triple Berry Smoothie

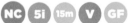

180 calories

Entire recipe (about 12 ounces): 180 calories, 2g total fat (0g sat fat), 152mg sodium, 25g carbs, 5.5g fiber, 15g sugars, 17.5g protein

1 cup frozen mixed berries
½ cup unsweetened vanilla almond milk
One 5.3-ounce container fat-free plain Greek yogurt
2 packets natural no-calorie sweetener, or more to taste
½ cup crushed ice

Blend ingredients until smooth.

MAKES 1 SERVING

HG FYI
Check the fruit's ingredients list to make sure no sugar's been added.

5-Minute Smoothies

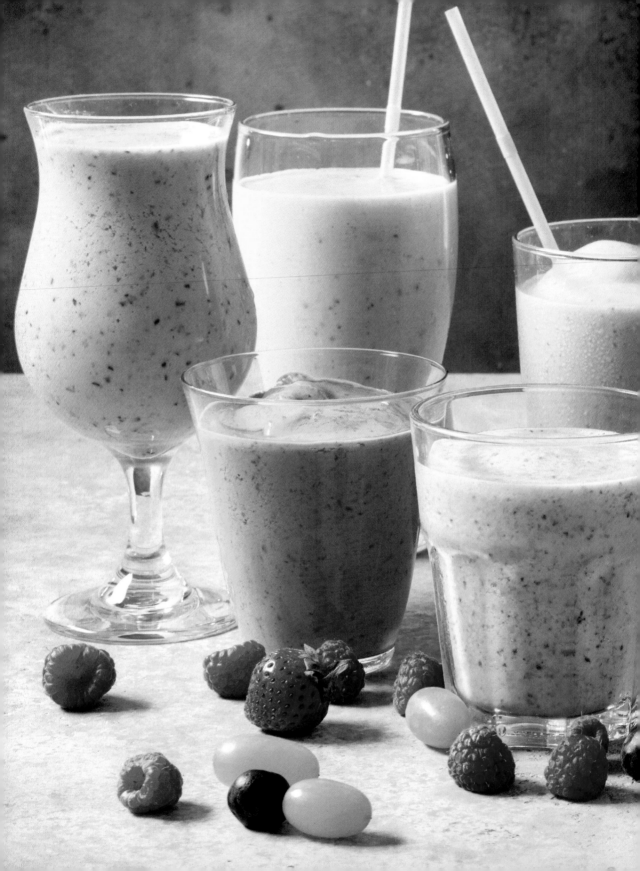

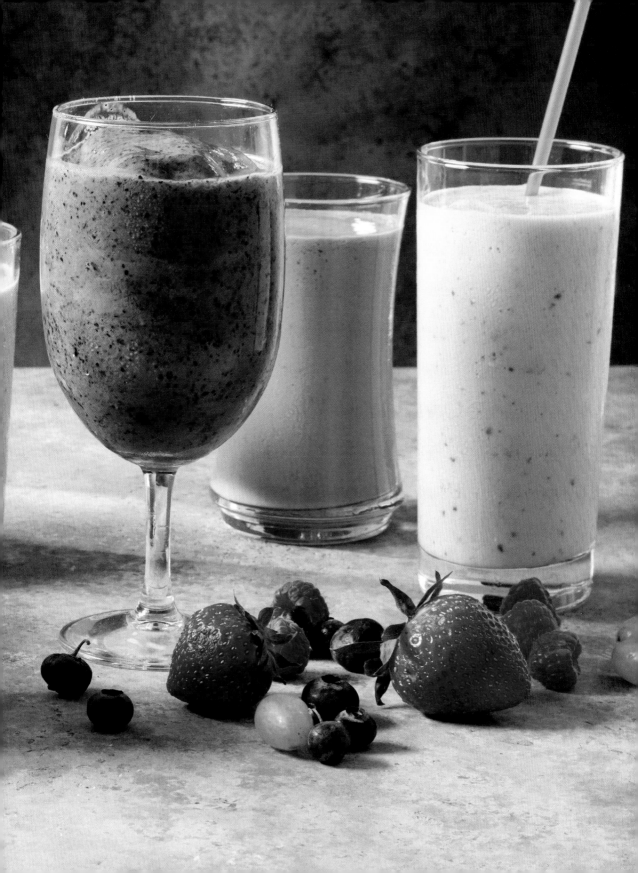

Cherry Vanilla Smoothie

243 calories

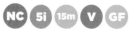 NC · 5i · 15m · V · GF

Entire recipe (about 12 ounces): 216 calories, 1.5g total fat (0g sat fat), 151mg sodium, 32g carbs, 3.5g fiber, 25g sugars, 17g protein

1 cup frozen dark sweet cherries
½ cup unsweetened vanilla almond milk
One 5.3-ounce container fat-free plain Greek yogurt
2 packets natural no-calorie sweetener, or more to taste
½ teaspoon vanilla extract

Blend ingredients until smooth.

MAKES 1 SERVING

Blueberry Coconut Smoothie

216 calories

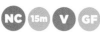 NC · 15m · V · GF

Entire recipe (about 14 ounces): 243 calories, 2g total fat (0g sat fat), 152mg sodium, 40.5g carbs, 5.5g fiber, 25.5g sugars, 17g protein

¾ cup frozen blueberries
½ cup frozen banana coins
½ cup unsweetened vanilla almond milk
One 5.3-ounce container fat-free plain Greek yogurt
2 packets natural no-calorie sweetener, or more to taste
½ teaspoon coconut extract

Blend ingredients until smooth.

MAKES 1 SERVING

HG Tip
Freeze ½-cup servings of banana coins in individual baggies for recipes like this. Easy freezy!

5-Minute Smoothies

Chocolate Raspberry Smoothie

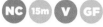

197 calories

Entire recipe (about 16 ounces): 197 calories, 2g total fat (<0.5g sat fat), 206mg sodium, 29g carbs, 7.5g fiber, 24.5g sugars, 18g protein

1 cup frozen raspberries
½ cup unsweetened vanilla almond milk
One 5.3-ounce container fat-free plain Greek yogurt
2 packets natural no-calorie sweetener, or more to taste
2 teaspoons light chocolate syrup
2 teaspoons unsweetened dark cocoa powder

Blend ingredients until smooth.

MAKES 1 SERVING

Pumpkin Apple Smoothie

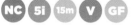

204 calories

Entire recipe (about 20 ounces): 204 calories, 1.5g total fat (0g sat fat), 154mg sodium, 31.5g carbs, 5.5g fiber, 21g sugars, 17.5g protein

1 cup chopped Fuji apple
½ cup unsweetened vanilla almond milk
One 5.3-ounce container fat-free plain Greek yogurt
⅓ cup canned pure pumpkin
2 packets natural no-calorie sweetener, or more to taste
¼ teaspoon cinnamon
⅛ teaspoon pumpkin pie spice
¾ cup crushed ice

Blend ingredients until smooth.

MAKES 1 SERVING

5-Minute Smoothies

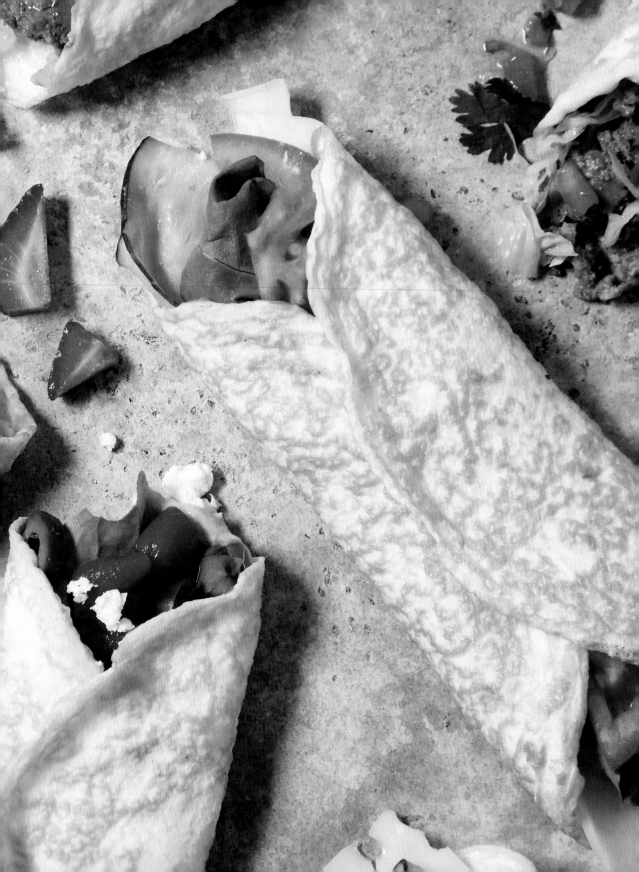

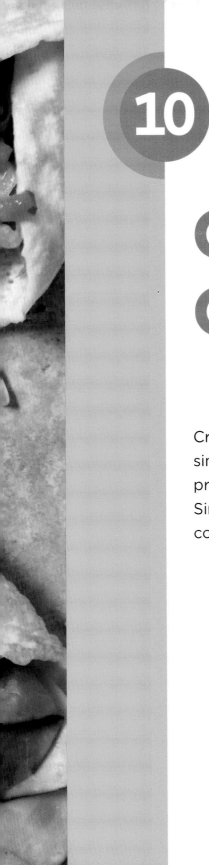

10

Quickie Crepes

Crepes may sound fancy, but mine are super simple to make. Bonus: They're PACKED with protein . . . Start with the Simple Savory or Simple Sweet Crepes, and then whip up the combos on the following pages!

Simple Savory Crepes

47 calories

½ cup (about 4 large) egg whites or fat-free liquid egg substitute

1½ tablespoons plain protein powder with about 100 calories per scoop

¼ teaspoon garlic powder

¼ teaspoon onion powder

1. In a medium bowl, whisk all ingredients until uniform.

2. Bring a 10-inch skillet sprayed with nonstick spray to medium heat. Pour half of the batter into the pan, quickly tilting the skillet in all directions to evenly coat the bottom. Cook until lightly browned, about 1½ minutes per side.

3. Repeat to make a second crepe.

MAKES 2 SERVINGS

Prep: 5 minutes

Cook: 10 minutes

You'll need: medium bowl, whisk, 10-inch skillet, nonstick spray

½ of recipe (1 crepe):
47 calories
<0.5g total fat
(0g sat fat)
114mg sodium
1.5g carbs
0g fiber
0.5g sugars
9g protein

Quickie Crepes

½ cup (about 4 large) egg whites or fat-free liquid egg substitute

1½ tablespoons plain protein powder with about 100 calories per scoop

1 packet natural no-calorie sweetener

¼ teaspoon vanilla extract

⅛ teaspoon cinnamon

1. In a medium bowl, whisk all ingredients until uniform.

2. Bring a 10-inch skillet sprayed with nonstick spray to medium heat. Pour half of the batter into the pan, quickly tilting the skillet in all directions to evenly coat the bottom. Cook until lightly browned, about 1½ minutes per side.

3. Repeat to make a second crepe.

MAKES 2 SERVINGS

49 calories

Prep: 5 minutes

Cook: 10 minutes

You'll need:
medium bowl, whisk, 10-inch skillet, nonstick spray

½ of recipe (1 crepe):
49 calories
<0.5g total fat
(0g sat fat)
114mg sodium
1.5g carbs
0g fiber
0.5g sugars
9g protein

HG Tip
Make a bunch of Sweet & Savory Crepes at once, store them in the fridge, and use throughout the week!

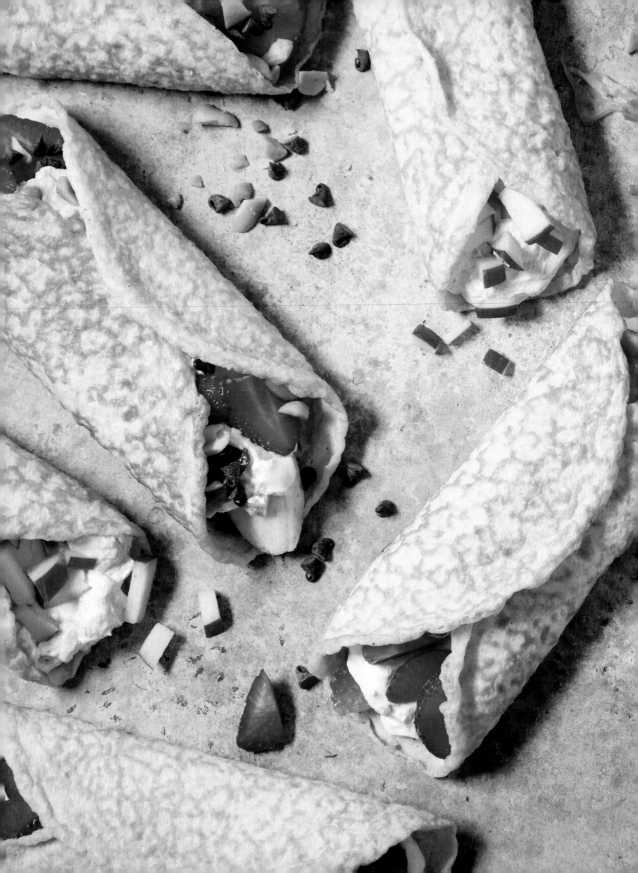

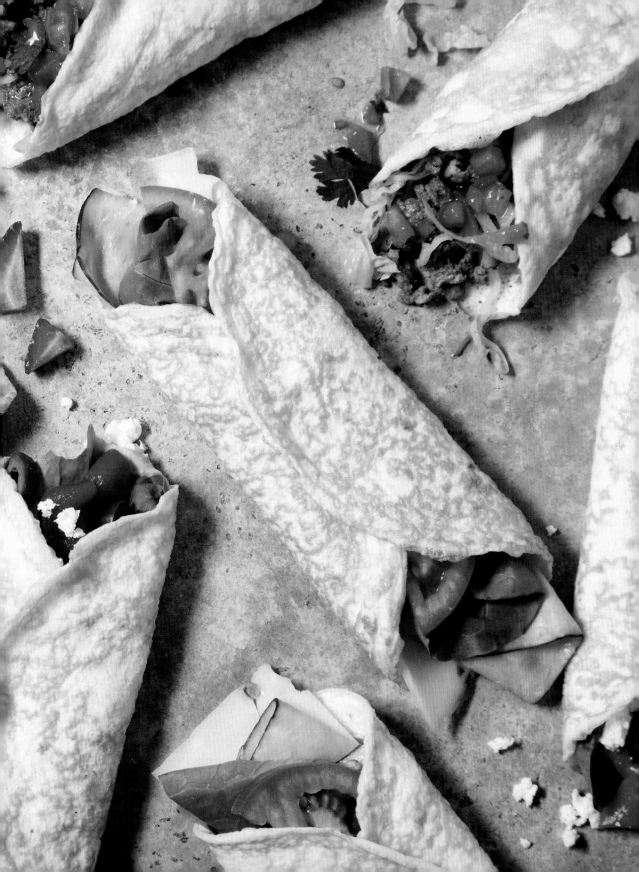

Ham & Swiss Crepes

137 calories

15m GF

½ of recipe (1 crepe): 137 calories, 3g total fat (1g sat fat), 552mg sodium, 5.5g carbs, 0.5g fiber, 3g sugars, 20g protein

2 Simple Savory Crepes, page 296
3 ounces (about 6 slices) reduced-sodium ham
1 slice reduced-fat Swiss cheese, sliced in half
2 slices tomato, halved
2 large lettuce leaves
2 teaspoons Dijon or honey mustard

Divide ingredients between crepes, and roll up crepes over the filling.

MAKES 2 SERVINGS

Southwestern Crepes

160 calories

15m GF

½ of recipe (1 crepe): 160 calories, 4.5g total fat (2.5g sat fat), 320mg sodium, 4g carbs, 0.5g fiber, 2g sugars, 23g protein

4 ounces extra-lean ground beef (at least 96% lean)
½ teaspoon taco seasoning
2 Simple Savory Crepes, page 296
½ cup shredded lettuce
2 tablespoons shredded reduced-fat cheddar cheese
2 tablespoons salsa
1 tablespoon light sour cream
1 tablespoon chopped fresh cilantro

Cook beef with taco seasoning. Divide lettuce and beef between crepes, and top with remaining ingredients. Roll up crepes over the filling.

MAKES 2 SERVINGS

Quickie Crepes

Hungry Girl FAST & Easy

131 calories

½ of recipe (1 crepe): 131 calories, 5g total fat (1.5g sat fat), 496mg sodium, 7.5g carbs, 0.5g fiber, 2.5g sugars, 11.5g protein

2 Simple Savory Crepes, page 296
2 tablespoons hummus
½ cup chopped jarred roasted red peppers packed in water, drained
2 tablespoons sliced Kalamata or black olives
2 tablespoons crumbled feta cheese
½ cup spinach

Divide ingredients between crepes, and roll up crepes over the filling.

MAKES 2 SERVINGS

Banana Split Crepes

215 calories

½ of recipe (1 crepe): 215 calories, 6g total fat (3.5g sat fat), 120mg sodium, 30g carbs, 3g fiber, 17.5g sugars, 11g protein

1 medium banana, halved lengthwise
2 Simple Sweet Crepes, page 297
1 teaspoon vanilla extract
½ cup natural light whipped topping
½ cup sliced strawberries
¼ ounce (about 1 tablespoon) chopped peanuts
2 teaspoons mini semisweet chocolate chips

Place a banana half on each crepe. Mix vanilla extract into whipped topping, and spoon over banana halves. Top with remaining ingredients, and roll up crepes over the filling.

MAKES 2 SERVINGS

Quickie Crepes

Apple Cinnamon Crepes

210 calories

15m **V** **GF**

½ of recipe (1 crepe): 210 calories, 8.5g total fat (6g sat fat), 264mg sodium, 18g carbs, 1g fiber, 11g sugars, 14g protein

½ cup natural light whipped topping
¼ cup light/reduced-fat cream cheese, room temperature
¼ cup fat-free plain Greek yogurt
2 packets natural no-calorie sweetener
1 teaspoon vanilla extract
¼ teaspoon cinnamon
2 Simple Sweet Crepes, page 297
½ cup finely chopped Fuji or Gala apple

Mix all ingredients except crepes and apple, and divide mixture between crepes. Top with apple, and roll up crepes over the filling.

MAKES 2 SERVINGS

½ of recipe (1 crepe): 206 calories, 8.5g total fat (6g sat fat), 342mg sodium, 17g carbs, 1g fiber, 10g sugars, 14.5g protein

206 calories

½ **cup natural light whipped topping**
¼ **cup light/reduced-fat cream cheese, room temperature**
¼ **cup fat-free plain Greek yogurt**
2 **packets natural no-calorie sweetener**
1 **teaspoon vanilla extract**
Dash salt
2 **Simple Sweet Crepes, page 297**
½ **cup chopped strawberries**

Mix all ingredients except crepes and strawberries, and divide mixture between crepes. Top with strawberries, and roll up crepes over the filling.

MAKES 2 SERVINGS

Quickie Crepes

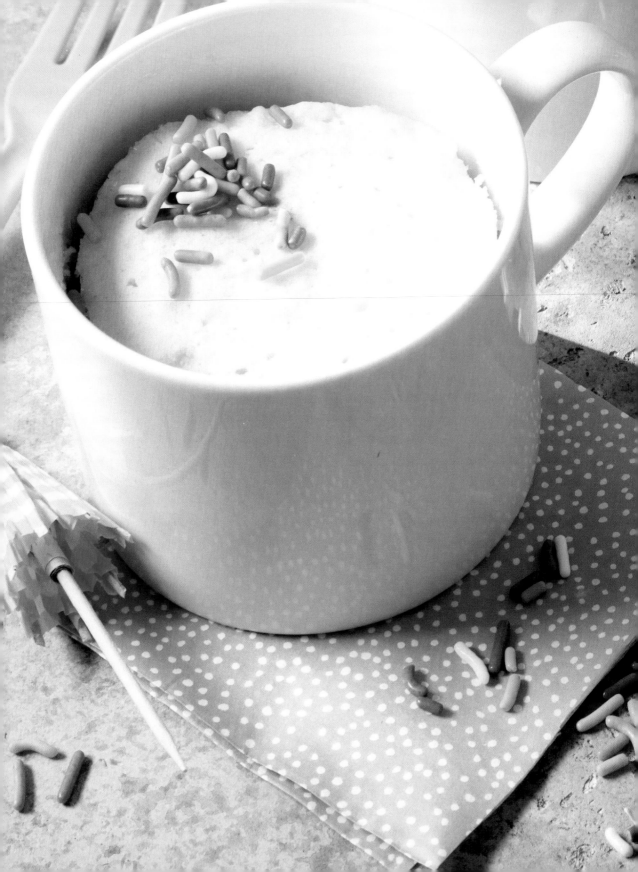

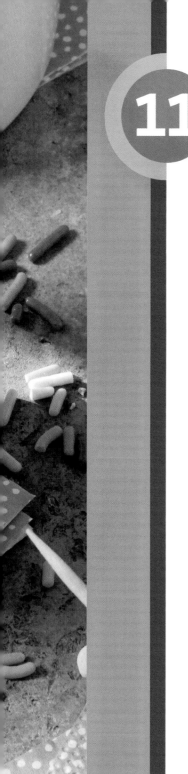

11

2-Ingredient Cake Mugs

Need a sweet treat in a flash? You're only two ingredients and a few minutes away from a cake for one. Grab a mug, and let's get going!

Orange Cloud Cake Mug

164 calories

Entire recipe: 164 calories, 0g total fat (0g sat fat), 339mg sodium, 37g carbs, <0.5g fiber, 27.5g sugars, 3.5g protein

¼ **cup angel food cake mix**
2 tablespoons mandarin orange segments packed in juice (not drained)

Spray a microwave-safe mug with nonstick spray. Add ingredients, and thoroughly mash and mix. Microwave for 1 minute and 15 seconds, or until set.

MAKES 1 SERVING

Yum Yum Chocolate Cake Mug

166 calories

Entire recipe: 166 calories, 3g total fat (1g sat fat), 332mg sodium, 34g carbs, 2.5g fiber, 18.5g sugars, 2.5g protein

¼ **cup devil's food cake or chocolate cake mix**
2 tablespoons canned pure pumpkin

Spray a microwave-safe mug with nonstick spray. Add ingredients and 1 tablespoon water. Thoroughly mix. (Batter will be THICK.) Microwave for 1 minute, or until set.

MAKES 1 SERVING

2-Ingredient Cake Mugs

Hungry Girl *FAST* & Easy

141 calories

Entire recipe: 141 calories, 1.5g total fat (1g sat fat), 292mg sodium, 31g carbs, 1g fiber, 16g sugars, 1g protein

¼ **cup confetti/rainbow cake mix**
2 **tablespoons no-calorie lemon-lime soda**

Spray a microwave-safe mug with nonstick spray. Add ingredients, and thoroughly mix. Microwave for 1 minute, or until set.

MAKES 1 SERVING

HG Tip

**All-natural cake mixes are gaining in popularity . . .
Check your local natural-foods store, or stock up online!**

2-Ingredient Cake Mugs

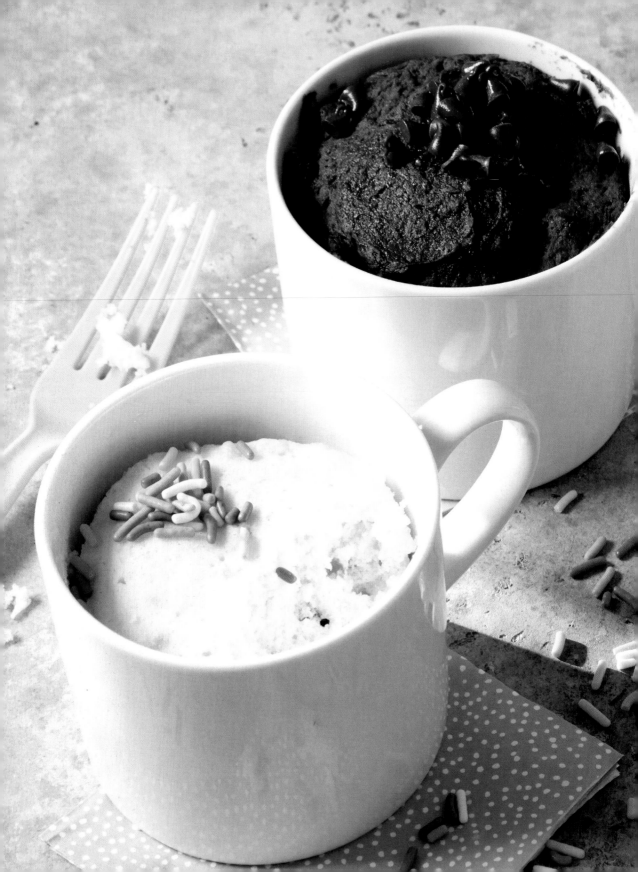

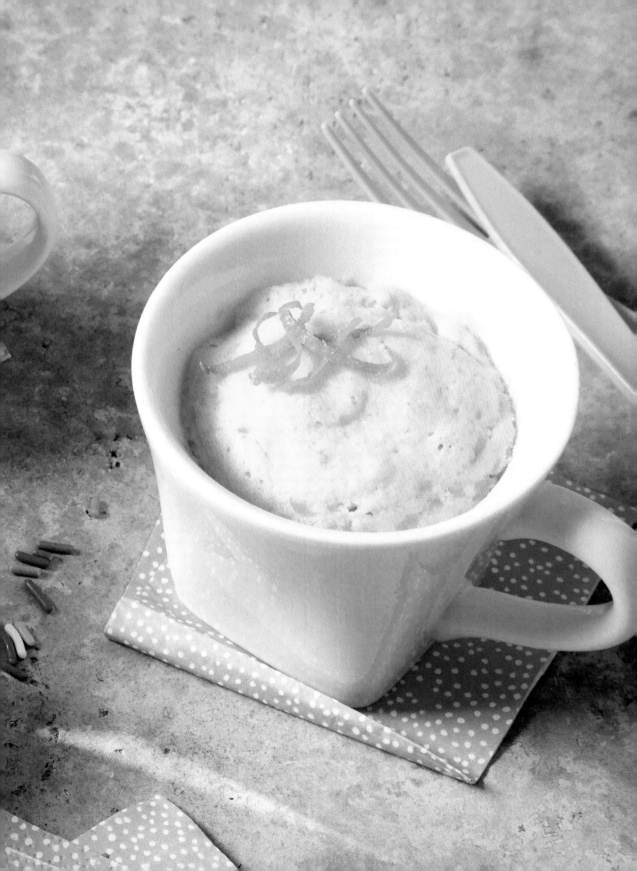

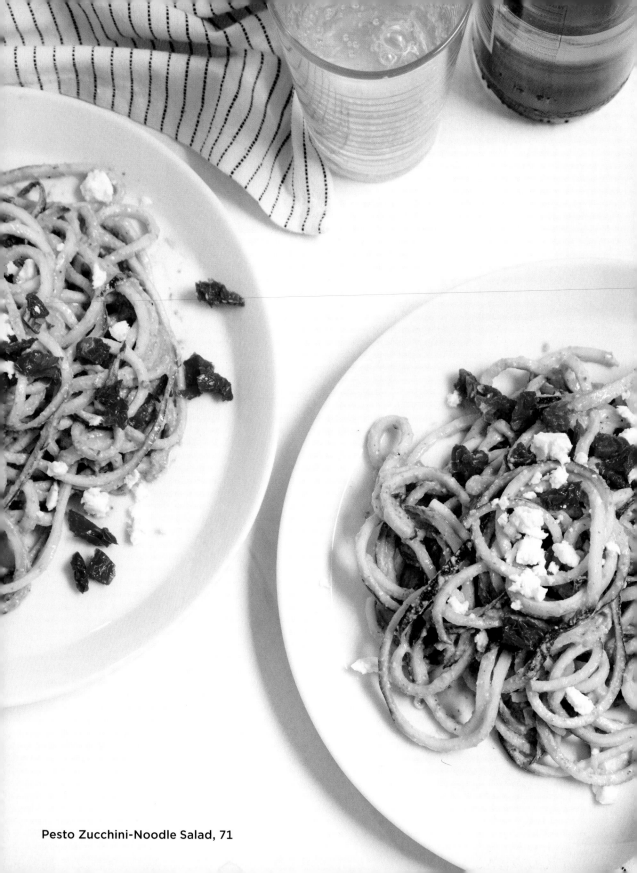

Pesto Zucchini-Noodle Salad, 71

12

Fast & Easy Kitchen Guides

Frozen riced cauliflower, a.k.a. cauliflower rice, works perfectly in recipes! No prep, already cooked, lasts for months in the freezer . . . What's not to love? Of course, if you'd prefer to use fresh cauliflower rice, I've got you covered.

How to Make Riced Cauliflower

Start with roughly chopped cauliflower florets, and pulse them in a blender until reduced to rice-size pieces. Don't overfill your blender . . . blend a cup or two at a time. You may need to stop and stir occasionally in order to finish the job.

How to Store Riced Cauliflower

Transfer your veggie rice to a large sealable airtight container, and refrigerate for up to five days. You can freeze it too!

How to Use Fresh Cauliflower Rice in These Recipes

Frozen cauliflower rice is precooked, so you'll need to cook your freshly riced cauliflower before adding it to a recipe. Just microwave it in a covered bowl for 2 minutes, or until soft. So easy!

HG FYI

A food processor doesn't work quite as well here— you could easily end up with cauliflower crumbs!

Riced Cauliflower Recipes

HG Tip
1 cup cauliflower florets = about ¾ cup cauliflower rice.
More helpful veggie stats await on page 331!

Fast & Easy Kitchen Guides

Spiralized Zucchini Guide

Several recipes in this cookbook call for spiralized zucchini . . . It's a perfect fast & easy pasta swap! DIY your spirals, or find them ready to go in both the fridge and freezer sections of the supermarket.

How to Spiralize Zucchini

All you need is a simple handheld veggie spiralizer. Typically, you can find one for less than $10 online or in stores. Holding the stem end, feed the zucchini into the blade, rotating to churn out the noodles. The noodles may be long, so give 'em a rough chop!

How to Store Spiralized Zucchini

Place your spirals in a large sealable airtight container, and refrigerate for up to five days. Spiralizing squash is a great weekend meal-prep activity!

How to Use Frozen Spirals in These Recipes

These recipes call for fresh spiralized veggies, but I enjoy frozen ones as well. They're so convenient and last for months in your freezer! Just heat them according to the package directions, and drain any excess water. For hot recipes, add them during the final minute or so of cooking, just long enough to make sure they're hot and well mixed.

HG Alternative
Use a basic veggie peeler! Peel the zucchini into thin strips, rotating it after each swipe of the peeler so the slices are uniform in size.

Fast & Easy Kitchen Guides

Spiralized Veggie Recipes

- Pesto Zucchini-Noodle Salad, page 71

- Ground Beef Stroganoff, page 95

- Garlic-Butter Shrimp with Squash Noodles, page 107

- Shrimp Pad Thai, page 111

- Zoodle Tofu Ramen, page 239

- Asian Style Shrimp & Zucchini Noodle Bowl, page 258

HG Tip
1 medium zucchini = about 8 ounces or 1½ cups spiralized zucchini.
Flip to page 331 for more produce tips and tricks!

Fast & Easy Kitchen Guides

Ground meat is great . . . Minimal prep, it cooks up quickly, and it's delicious in everything—even as a pizza crust. (See page 151 for proof!) The recipes in this book call for extra-lean ground meats, but if you can't find those or just prefer the taste of meat with a higher fat content, here's everything you need to know about swapping . . .

Ground Beef

What to look for: Extra-lean ground beef (at least 96% lean)

How it tastes: Super flavorful and juicy

Lean alternative (at least 92% lean): Add 25 calories and 3g total fat per 4-ounce serving

Ground Turkey

What to look for: Extra-lean ground turkey (at least 98% lean)

How it tastes: Not as flavorful or moist as beef, but the best bang for your calorie buck

Lean alternative (at least 93% lean): Add 40 calories and 5.5g total fat per 4-ounce serving

Ground Chicken

What to look for: Extra-lean ground chicken (at least 98% lean)

How it tastes: Similar to extra-lean ground turkey . . . Best with plenty of seasoning

Lean alternative (at least 93% lean): Add 15 calories and 4.5g total fat per 4-ounce serving

Vegetarian Bonus: Meatless Crumbles

Prefer a plant-based option? Swap in 1 cup of crumbles for every 4 ounces of ground meat. Most beef-style crumbles are fully cooked, so simply add them toward the end of the recipe's cook time, and cook until hot.

Ground Meat at a Glance

Extra-Lean Ground Beef
4 ounces = 145 calories, 5g total fat, 23.5g protein

Extra-Lean Ground Turkey
4 ounces = 120 calories, 2g total fat, 27g protein

Extra-Lean Ground Chicken
4 ounces = 135 calories, 1.5g total fat, 25.5g protein

Meatless Crumbles
1 cup = 125 calories, 2.5g total fat, 20g protein

Ingredient Swaps Made Simple

These recipes are delicious as is, but that doesn't mean you can't mix things up a little! Here are our favorite swaps in several categories. Get inspired, and feel free to use these foods interchangeably . . .

Salad Greens

romaine lettuce, mixed greens, arugula, spinach, kale

Riced Veggies

riced cauliflower, riced broccoli

Veggie Noodles

spiralized zucchini, spiralized yellow squash, spiralized carrots, broccoli slaw, coleslaw mix, bean sprouts

Quick-Cooking Veggies

mushrooms, zucchini, yellow squash, tomatoes, spinach, kale, cauliflower, bell peppers, onions, green beans

Slow-Cooking Veggies

Brussels sprouts, eggplant, asparagus, butternut squash, cauliflower, broccoli

Frozen Veggies

stir-fry vegetables, petite mixed veggies, broccoli & cauliflower

Meat, Poultry & Seafood

lean flank steak, chicken breast, fully cooked chicken sausage, skinless turkey breast, shrimp, scallops, salmon, cod, tuna

Ground Meat

extra-lean chicken, turkey, or beef (at least 96% lean)

Recipe nutritional info may vary when making swaps.

Fast & Easy Kitchen Guides

Make It Vegan: Plant-Based Swaps!

Most of these recipes can be made vegan with a few key ingredient swaps, and these substitutes are easy to find! Here's what you need to know . . .

Cheese

From slices to shreds, vegan cheese has come a long way. The taste, texture, and meltability are better than ever! It's commonly made from tofu, soy, or nuts.

Stats to Look For: 60 calories per slice; 80 calories per ¼ cup shreds

Find It: In the refrigerated tofu section or with the regular cheese

Eggs

For frittatas, crepes, and more, vegan egg substitute is the perfect choice. The liquid kind is made from soy; powdered options are often made with potato starch. For baked goods and meatballs, use flaxseed meal (a.k.a. ground flaxseed). Simply mix 1 tablespoon with 3 tablespoons water for each egg (or ¼ cup egg whites) called for in the recipe.

Stats to Look For: 70 calories per ¼ cup liquid or powder; 35 calories per tablespoon of flax

Find It: In the baking aisle, refrigerated tofu section, or egg aisle

> ### HG Tip
> **For breaded & baked recipes dredged in egg to make the crumbs stick, use a dairy-free sauce instead. Think BBQ sauce, mustard . . . Flavorful and vegan friendly!**

Ground Meat

Soy crumbles are one of my favorite finds. They're great in tacos, stir-frys, chili, and more. Use 1 cup crumbles for every 4 ounces of ground meat. Prepare them according to the package directions, and add them toward the end of the recipe.

Stats to Look For: 60–80 calories per ½ cup

Find It: In the freezer aisle or refrigerated section, near the other meatless swaps

Chicken Breast

Reach for precooked veggie chik'n strips, made from soy and wheat protein. If you're not feeling a faux chicken, choose tofu or tempeh. Tofu is perfect for chicken-style nuggets. If you prefer a soy-free protein, choose seitan (made from wheat protein).

Stats to Look For: 120–140 calories per 3-ounce serving

Find It: In the freezer aisle or the refrigerated tofu section

Deli Meat

Yes, there are plant-based deli slices! They're made with ingredients like soy protein, bean flour, wheat gluten, and tofu. Perfect in salads, sandwiches, and more.

Stats to Look For: 70–100 calories per 2-ounce serving

Find It: In the refrigerated tofu section

Chicken Sausage

Plant-based sausage is a super swap. It's made with things like pea protein, wheat gluten, and potato flour, so check the labels if you're vegan and gluten free.

Stats to Look For: 140–170 calories per 3-ounce link

Find It: In the refrigerated tofu section

Tuna

Tuna from plants? It exists! Common ingredients include pea protein, potato starch, beans, and seaweed powder.

Stats to Look For: 40–60 calories per 2-ounce serving

Find It: In the canned goods aisle, near the regular tuna

Mayonnaise

Sure, you could just use mustard, but vegan mayo is another smart swap. It's made with things like oil, bean broth, soybean oil, and bean protein for that signature tangy taste.

Stats to Look For: 70–90 calories per tablespoon

Find It: In the refrigerated tofu section

> **HG Alternative**
> If you'd prefer a veggie-only protein, try beans, lentils, or edamame instead.

Fast & Easy Kitchen Guides

Cream Cheese

Yes, even cream cheese can be made without dairy. The vegan versions often use coconut, potato protein, pea protein, and nuts to get that signature texture.

Stats to Look For: 60–90 calories per 2-tablespoon serving

Find It: With the dairy items, or near the refrigerated tofu

Butter

Look for butter substitutes made from plant-based oils and pea protein. Or just trade your butter for a small amount of olive, coconut, or avocado oil (which are higher in calories).

Stats to Look For: 60–90 calories per tablespoon

Find It: In the butter section or baking aisle

Yogurt

The dairy aisle is full of delicious, rich, creamy plant-based options, made from soy, almond milk, and coconut milk. There's even Greek-style dairy-free yogurt! Stock up on the plain kind for ultimate versatility.

Stats to Look For: 100–120 calories per single-serving container

Find It: In the yogurt section

Recipe nutritional info may vary when making swaps.

What to Do with Leftover Ingredients

So you bought a can of tomatoes, but only used half a cup? Here are some simple recipe ideas and storage solutions for common leftover ingredients . . .

Avocado

Refrigerate: 3–4 days once cut

Freeze: 3–6 months for mashed avocados

> **HG Tip**
> **Add a little lemon juice and tightly wrap to prevent browning.**

Recipe Ideas

- Mash and mix with Greek yogurt or salsa for a two-ingredient dip

- Spread onto whole-wheat bread or high-fiber crackers, and sprinkle with everything bagel seasoning

- Add to salads and sandwiches

Canned Crushed Tomatoes

Refrigerate: 5–7 days once opened

Freeze: 3 months

Recipe Ideas

- Mix with Italian seasoning and use like marinara sauce

- Add beans, veggies, and seasonings for a quick chili

- Mix with cream cheese & taco seasoning for a fiesta dip

Broth

Refrigerate: 4–5 days once opened

Freeze: 6 months

Recipe Ideas

- Use in place of water when steaming veggies (so much flavor!)
- Add veggies and freeze for anytime soup
- Enjoy on its own—it's a sippable snack!

Canned Beans

Refrigerate: 3–4 days once opened

Freeze: 1–2 months

Recipe Ideas

- Toss with seasonings and a little oil, and roast until crispy
- Add to egg scrambles and omelettes
- Give your salads a plant-based protein boost

Marinara Sauce

Refrigerate: 5–10 days once opened

Freeze: 6 months

Recipe Ideas

- Use in place of salsa or ketchup on your morning eggs
- Toss with spiralized veggies for a simple pasta swap
- Spread on a light English muffin, top with mozzarella, and broil. Hello, mini pizzas!

Fresh Veggies

Refrigerate: varies, best to use within a week

Freeze: 3–12 months

Recipe Ideas

- Whip up a green smoothie (add frozen fruit for texture and natural sweetness)
- Cook with teriyaki sauce for easy stir-fry
- Make a mix & match salad. (Don't forget the dressings starting on page 264.)

HG FYI
Don't freeze vegetables with a high-water content. These include lettuce, cabbage, celery, and cucumbers.

Time-Saving Tips from the Test Kitchen

Here are some tried & true tips straight out of Hungryland to save you (even more) time & energy in your kitchen!

Before You Start . . .

Stock your fridge with recipe-ready ingredients

Cut veggies, chopped lettuce, ready-to-cook shrimp, and chicken cutlets . . . all staples in Hungry Girl recipes. Store them in airtight containers so they stay fresh.

Preheat the oven

It always seems to take longer than you think it will! Do this before you even begin to prep your ingredients.

Read the recipe in its entirety

It might sound obvious, but this can make following a recipe as you go much easier.

Pull out all your ingredients.

Measure them out, too, and you'll fly through the recipe process.

Set out your cooking supplies

Just look for the words "You'll Need" on the recipe page to find out what they are.

Along the Way . . .

Clean as you go

Keep a garbage can nearby, and tidy up between recipe steps. Load the dishwasher, wipe down the counters, put away extra ingredients . . . You'll be amazed at how much you can get done before dinner even hits the plate!

Pull out containers for leftovers

Who says you can't be too prepared? Not our test kitchen! Flip to the Meal-Prep Guide on the next page for more tips & tricks . . .

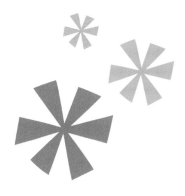

Fast & Easy Kitchen Guides

Nothing is faster, easier, or (in the case of this book!) more delicious than leftovers. Many of the recipes in this cookbook give you 4+ servings, and you can easily multiply the single-serving recipes. So I recommend making room in your fridge and freezer for make-ahead meals . . .

Refrigeration 101

Hold off on the fresh toppings

Save things like salsa, sour cream, and salad dressing for day-of topping off . . .

Divide and cool

Divide the dish into equal-size servings, using microwave-safe containers with airtight lids. This way, you'll have perfect portions that cool quickly, thaw nicely, and reheat in no time.

Into the fridge

Great news! Almost ALL the recipes in this book will stay fresh for several days in the refrigerator.

Reheat and eat!

Remove the lid or vent it before placing the container in the microwave. Then heat the dish for a minute at a time (less for smaller items), until it reaches your desired temperature.

Freezy Does It

Pack it up

Add individual servings to freezer-friendly containers with airtight lids.

Plan ahead

The best way to thaw is in the fridge overnight. Then simply reheat when you're ready to eat.

The microwave method . . .

If you forgot to thaw your food overnight, no problem. Pop it into the microwave, and hit the defrost button. Check on it every minute or two, stirring or rotating as needed.

What to freeze

Stir-Frys • Sheet-Pan Meals • Soups • Stews

What NOT to freeze

Salads • Slaws • Veggie Noodle Dishes

Hungry Girl recipes call for most vegetables by measurement (like 1 cup sliced onion) as opposed to number (like 1 onion). It's more exact, which means better recipe results. But if you need a little help when you hit the supermarket, this handy chart has you covered . . .

Bell Pepper

1 large bell pepper = about 1 cup chopped or sliced

Onion

1 large onion = 2–3 cups chopped or sliced

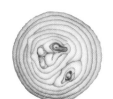

Avocado

1 medium avocado = about 4 ounces (½ cup chopped or 1 cup sliced)

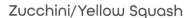

Zucchini/Yellow Squash

1 medium squash = 1–1½ cups chopped or spiralized

Tomatoes

1 medium tomato = ½ cup chopped

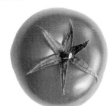

Mushrooms

8 ounces mushrooms = 2–3 cups chopped or sliced

Bagged Greens

- One 12-ounce bag broccoli slaw = about 4 cups

- One bag coleslaw mix (14–16 ounces) = 8–10 cups

- One bag lettuce (9–12 ounces) = about 6–8 cups

Never hit the supermarket without a plan . . . Here's an aisle-by-aisle list of common fast & easy ingredients for these recipes and beyond!

Dairy & Dairy Swaps

- reduced-fat cheese (both shredded & sliced)
- crumbled feta cheese
- grated Parmesan cheese
- light/reduced-fat cream cheese
- light/low-fat ricotta cheese
- fat-free plain Greek yogurt
- eggs, liquid egg whites, and/or fat-free liquid egg substitute
- unsweetened vanilla almond milk
- light sour cream
- whipped butter
- light mayonnaise

Meat & Seafood

Poultry

- skinless chicken breast (both raw & cooked)
- fully cooked chicken sausage
- extra-lean ground chicken or turkey (at least 98% lean)
- sliced skinless turkey breast (reduced-sodium)

Beef

- extra-lean ground beef (at least 96% lean)
- lean flank steak

Pork

- lean pork tenderloin
- boneless pork chops
- sliced ham (reduced-sodium)

Bacon

- center-cut bacon or turkey bacon
- precooked crumbled bacon

Seafood

- tilapia, tuna, salmon & other fish fillets
- shrimp
- scallops
- crab (real or imitation)
- smoked salmon
- canned or pouched albacore tuna packed in water

Produce

Bagged Produce

- chopped lettuce
- spinach
- coleslaw mix
- broccoli slaw

More Fresh Veggies

- bell peppers
- onions
- mushrooms
- zucchini & yellow squash
- tomatoes

Frozen Vegetables

- stir-fry vegetables
- sweet corn kernels
- riced cauliflower (or DIY)
- spiralized zucchini (or DIY)
- broccoli & cauliflower

Fresh Fruit

- apples
- berries
- oranges

Frozen Fruit

- strawberries
- mango chunks
- peach slices

. . . and MORE fruits and veggies!

Canned & Jarred Foods

- tomatoes (crushed, stewed & diced)
- chicken, beef & vegetable broth
- beans (black, kidney, garbanzo, refried & more)
- sliced water chestnuts
- pineapple packed in juice
- mandarin orange segments packed in juice

Sauces, Salad Dressings & Condiments

- light salad dressings
- vinegar (balsamic, rice & more)
- BBQ sauce with 45 calories or less per 2-tablespoon serving
- mustard (yellow, honey & Dijon)
- ketchup
- powdered peanut butter
- low-sugar fruit preserves & jam
- marinara sauce with 70 calories or less per 2-tablespoon serving
- salsa
- reduced-sodium/lite soy sauce
- thick teriyaki sauce or marinade
- sweet chili sauce
- enchilada sauce (red & green)
- chicken or turkey gravy

Baking Products & Pantry Staples

- old-fashioned oats
- whole-wheat flour
- panko bread crumbs
- almonds
- pistachios
- 6-inch corn tortillas
- bagged sun-dried tomatoes (not packed in oil)
- sweetened dried cranberries
- protein powder with about 100 calories per scoop
- mini semisweet chocolate chips
- unsweetened cocoa powder
- nonstick cooking spray
- olive oil
- natural no-calorie sweetener packets
- natural no-calorie granulated sweetener
- everything bagel seasoning
- taco seasoning
- chili seasoning
- jarred chopped garlic (refrigerate once opened)

Visit hungry-girl.com/fast&easy for a printable version of this list!

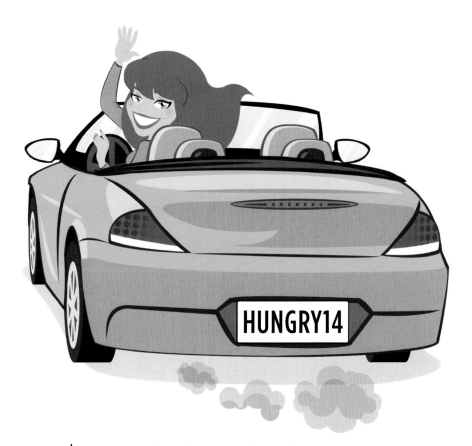

Wow! I guess that's it. If you're reading this you've either finished reading the whole book or flipped to the end for some reason. I think you need to go back and start flagging all the recipes you want to try. (I highly recommend the Chicken Cordon Bleu Stir-Fry on p. 76 and the Cheeseburger Heaven on p. 219, but they're all great!) And for more healthy recipes, plus food finds, tips, tricks, hacks & more, sign up for my free daily emails at hungry-girl.com.

'Til next time . . . Chew the right thing!

Lisa :)

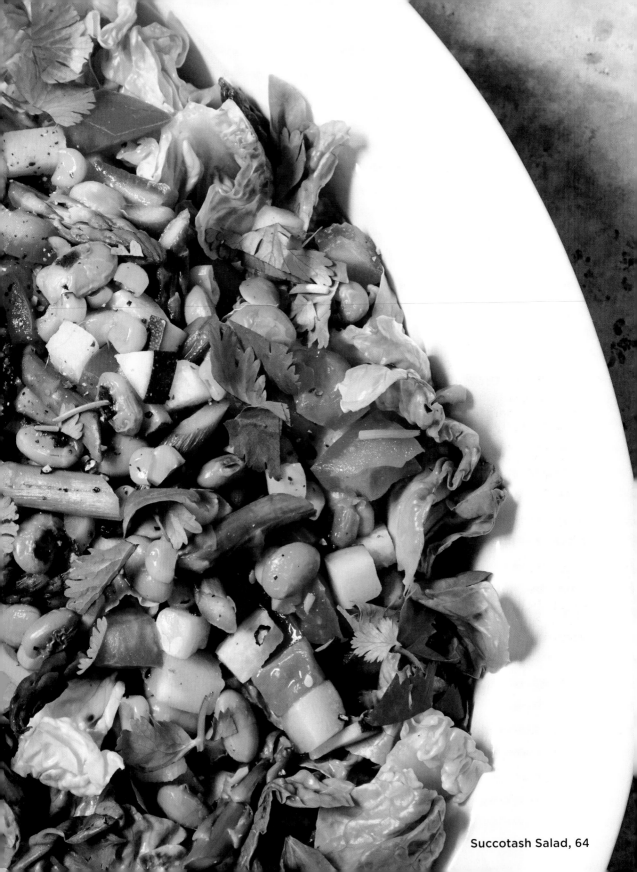

Succotash Salad, 64

Index

P